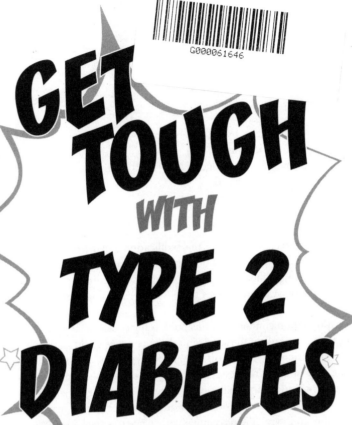

GET TOUGH

WITH

TYPE 2
DIABETES

Master your diabetes

DR DAVID LEVY

BOOKS

Hammersmith Health Books
London, UK

First published in 2018 by Hammersmith Health Books – an imprint of
Hammersmith Books Limited
4/4A Bloomsbury Square, London WC1A 2RP, UK
www.hammersmithbooks.co.uk

The information contained in this book is for educational purposes
only. It is the result of the study and the experience of the author. Whilst
the information and advice offered are believed to be true and accurate
at the time of going to press, neither the author nor the publisher can
accept any legal responsibility or liability for any errors or omissions
that may have been made or for any adverse effects which may occur as
a result of following the recommendations given herein. Always consult
a qualified medical practitioner if you have any concerns regarding your
health.

British Library Cataloguing in Publication Data: A CIP record of this
book is available from the British Library.

Print ISBN 978-1-78161-108-1
Ebook ISBN 978-1-78161-109-8

Commissioning editor: Georgina Bentliff
Designed and typeset by: Julie Bennett of Bespoke Publishing Ltd
Cover design by: Sylvia Kwan
Index: Dr Laurence Errington
Production: Helen Whitehorn of Path Projects Ltd
Printed and bound by: TJ International, UK

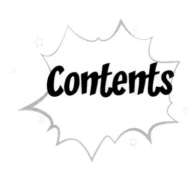

Contents

About the author

Dr David Levy was Consultant Physician in the Gillian Hanson Centre for Diabetes and Endocrinology, Whipps Cross University Hospital, London, UK and Hon Senior Lecturer at Queen Mary University of London, UK, until December 2014. He is still in active clinical practice, specialising in diabetes and endocrinology, and is the author of many books for healthcare professionals, including *Practical Diabetes Care* (4th edition, 2018), *Type 1 Diabetes* (2nd edition, 2016) and *The Hands-on Guide to Diabetes Care in Hospital* (2015), reflecting his interest in all aspects of clinical diabetes care.

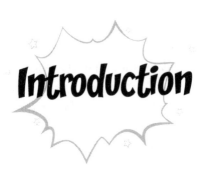

Introduction

Having Type 2 diabetes is tough. This book acknowledges that it's tough, but it's even tougher for Type 2s if they are continually bombarded by myths based on a misunderstanding of what Type 2 actually is. The prime myth is that Type 2 is caused by eating too much sugar, which then causes high blood glucose levels. It's tougher still when instructions about treatment come at us from all sides (for example, that treating Type 2 means stopping eating sugar, and if that doesn't work, then medication is needed, and eventually probably insulin – all inaccurate statements).

These simple tales about Type 2 never really made much sense, yet they continue to be told, believed and acted on. But over the past 20 years we've come to understand much more about the underlying causes of Type 2, and at last we're beginning to see proper scientific studies that take this new understanding and translate it – with great success, as we'll see – into treatments that are logical and therefore work. There is now clear trial evidence that, with admittedly rather tough interventions involving substantial weight loss, Type 2 can be reversed, and at last we can start thinking about managing the condition without the need for ever more blood glucose-lowering drugs. High blood glucose is the end result of Type 2 diabetes, not its cause.

Blood glucose is only one partner in the damage caused by Type 2 diabetes, and in fact it isn't as important as we once thought in the development of serious diabetes complications. It's abundantly clear that high blood pressure and abnormal cholesterol levels are at least as important in the heart attacks, strokes and kidney disease that are the most devastating long-term complications of diabetes. With careful and evidence-based lifestyle changes we can make real inroads, not only into high glucose levels but high blood pressure, with clear short- and long-term benefits. Cholesterol levels can be helped by careful attention to diet, though the high vascular risk of Type 2 means that medication is normally needed.

Diet and weight control are central to the day-to-day management of Type 2, and I discuss some of the newer ideas (see Chapter 5). That means getting tough on the latest 'superfoods', sadly none of which has been shown to improve blood glucose levels or reduce serious complications (see page 83). I also discuss the lessons to be learned from major clinical studies of diets. These include the Mediterranean approach, which reduces the risk of heart attacks, and possibly of cancer, and the lower-carbohydrate diet, which for many people is a more sustainable way of controlling weight than the traditional high-carbohydrate, low-saturated fat diet, which is coming under increased pressure from evidence (and, like the idea of sugar 'causing' Type 2 diabetes, was never really convincing).

Specific kinds of exercise and activity are important in many aspects of diabetes, although they don't have the same dramatic short-term effect as diet and weight loss. The evidence for the long-term benefits of exercise is distressingly thin, but regular moderate or vigorous exercise very likely reduces most of the complications of long-term diabetes, including premature death. We mustn't ignore the compelling evidence on activity and its important beneficial effects on general health, including perhaps postponing the frailty of later life.

Type 2 mostly affects people in middle age, and increasingly they are growing old gracefully with diabetes, because the complications that used to limit life expectancy are much less common than when I started working in diabetes in the 1980s. For that reason, Type 2 in older people is becoming a sub-specialty in its own right, because managing diabetes in later life requires an even more sensitive and careful approach than in younger people: kids with Type 1 diabetes need specialist paediatricians, so why shouldn't older Type 2s have their own experts?

Finally, it doesn't matter how much whiz-bang technology and clever new drugs there are, if you're depressed or distressed by your diabetes, everything will be more of a burden and less effective, so psychological approaches to Type 2 diabetes are tackled in Chapter 13. I feel a bit bad about this – it should, of course, be the first chapter – and if this little book ever comes to a revision, psychology may well come right at the beginning.

Ten years ago I wrote my first book for people with Type 2 and their carers, and at the time it seemed quite easy. The process was inadvertently helped by my publisher at the time thinking that the preliminary draft I sent him was the very final version, and he duly sent off my first thoughts for publication. Nobody noticed. In addition, back in 2007 we had very little evidence for the benefits of non-drug treatments, and too much of the book was devoted to current and upcoming medicines. Around the same time, some of the drugs turned out to have unexpected and severe side-effects, and since then I have become generally less enthusiastic about drug treatments, while recognising that when used carefully and sensitively they are, of course, extremely valuable. But we must always try to minimise the use of medication, and there is a separate chapter (page 98) on how to approach this – with caution, of course, professional support, naturally, but with some optimism.

Former colleagues at Whipps Cross University Hospital helped me to think through many of the topics covered in this book, and my current colleagues, especially Carin Hume and Una Vince at The London Diabetes Centre, have continued my education. Timo Pilgram, librarian at Whipps Cross, sourced references and scanned obscure medical niches of the internet, as he has done for all my recent diabetes books. My wife Laura scanned obscure culinary corners of the internet to maintain my food interest while writing, and helped with the sections on practical aspects of diet, especially the Mediterranean approach, which we aim to sample at least twice a year in countries where it originated. Carrying out scientific research is tough for authors.

Georgina Bentliff, publisher of Hammersmith Health Books, helped a great deal with the concept of the book. She commissioned it, cajoled me over deadlines – no toughness there, of course – and she and her team scrutinised the manuscript for evidence of plonky medical-speak, the clinical equivalent of management-speak or politician-speak. You know the kind of thing: 'the limited results from this prospective cohort study indicate that there may be some evidence for the increased efficacy of drug A compared with drug B, though further and larger trials are needed to confirm these preliminary findings …' If any similar horrors remain, blame me. It may be gently advancing age, but I've been amazed how difficult it was to write this book for non-medical people compared with my textbooks for professionals. I've never had to consign so many drafts to the electronic black-hole by activating the 'delete' button. Although we're trying to get tough with diabetes, no author should increase the difficulty for people with Type 2 by using indecipherable language, so let me or Georgina know if I could have done better.

David Levy
January 2018

How to use this book

A note on numbers and units

Blood glucose is measured in mmol/l ['milly-mole per litre']. Many countries use a different measurement – milligrams per decilitre (mg/dl). To convert mmol/l to mg/dl, multiply by 18.

Blood pressure is measured everywhere in mm Hg (millimetres of mercury), a reference to the old days when all pressures, including atmospheric pressure, were measured with a column of liquid mercury. Mercury, highly poisonous, hasn't been used in blood pressure equipment for many years, but the traditional unit remains.

Glycated haemoglobin (abbreviated to HbA_{1c} or A1C) indicates how high glucose levels have been over the previous six to eight weeks. It's not simply an average of blood glucose levels, but a completely different measurement, so it's not measured in mmol/l or mg/dl, although there are ways of estimating average blood glucose measurements from it. Ever since this ingenious measurement was introduced at the beginning of the 1980s, it has been reported as a percentage (%), usually in the range 6 to 10%, and that is how most people with diabetes remember it. Starting in 2011, a different measurement was introduced (mmol/mol, usually in the range 55 to 100). Because the percentage measurements were so familiar, many countries opted to continue reporting HbA_{1c} using both systems, so that healthcare professionals and people with diabetes can choose to use the units they are most familiar with. Unfortunately, in the UK the percentage reporting units were abolished around 2011, so HbA_{1c} is reported by NHS laboratories only in the new units.

Many internet sites have a simple HbA_{1c} converter. I usually Google 'convert HbA_{1c}' and go to the link with the excellent website Diabetes.co.uk (full web address is www.diabetes.co.uk/hba1c-units-converter.html).

For readers wanting to know more about this change in units, I wrote an article in 2013 discussing HbA_{1c} measurements and disputing the wisdom of the UK decision to permit only the 'new' reporting units (mmol/mol): 'HbA_{1c}: changing units, changing minds – mission accomplished?' in the *British Journal of Diabetes & Vascular Disease*.[1]

References and further reading

In each chapter I have included a few references to major studies published in medical journals together with a few websites. Wherever possible I have chosen references you can download in full text form for free. The easiest way to do this is to go to the website of the USA National Library of Medicine – www.PubMed.gov. In the search box enter the eight-digit PubMed number I have given at the end of the reference. This will bring up the 'abstract' of the paper – a short summary of its aims, methods, results and conclusions. If you'd like to see the full paper, follow the link indicated by 'Free full text' at the end of the abstract or 'Full Text Links' on the right of the screen.

Every medical research paper published in academic journals over the past 50 years is included in PubMed (and journals are progressively referencing historical material as far back as the 1920s), so in addition to looking up the references in this book, you can use it to research any medical topic you're interested in. Type your words of interest in the search box. Because PubMed contains *every* medical reference, if you look for papers on 'Type 2 diabetes', it will deliver about 150,000 possibilities, which might keep you occupied for a little while. Narrow your search – for example, 'Type 2 diabetes cardiac rehabilitation' yields about 140 references, with the most recently published papers first. If you click on 'Review' on the left of the screen, only articles summarising the current state of knowledge will be shown. Clicking on 'Free full text' will bring up only full-text articles that are available at no charge. PubMed is scientific and designed for doctors and medical scientists so the material is not always friendly to read, and contains lots of abbreviations which are not always spelt out. But everything quoted in PubMed is 'peer reviewed' – that is, scrutinised carefully by independent doctors and scientists – so, unlike the output of the usual search engines, it is generally trustworthy.

An example of an historical reference available in PubMed is the following short article of personal memories written by Charles Best in 1942, a year after the death of his colleague Frederick Banting in an air crash at the age of 49. Their initial experimental work was done in 1921 during a hot Toronto summer, when they isolated insulin and used it first to treat dogs who had been made diabetic by removing the pancreas. Insulin was first used in humans at the beginning of 1922.

Best CH. Reminiscences of the researches which led to the discovery of insulin. *Canadian Medical Association Journal* 1942; 47(5): 398-400. PubMed reference number 20322601. Free full text (www.ncbi.nlm.nih.gov/pmc/articles/ PMC1827503/pdf/canmedaj01696-0079.pdf)

The story of the discovery is described in detail in this book:

Bliss, Michael (2007). *The Discovery of Insulin*. Chicago, US: University of Chicago Press.

The wider history of diabetes is covered in this elegant little book, written by an eminent diabetes consultant:

Tattersall, Robert (2010). *Diabetes: The Biography* (Biographies of Disease). Oxford, UK: Oxford University Press.

Chapter 1

Understanding Type 2

Key points

- Type 2 is defined as blood glucose levels above a particular level.
- High blood glucose is only the final outcome of a pathway that originates in a complex package of abnormalities in several organs.
- The main abnormalities are in the liver and pancreas.
- In Type 2 the liver overproduces glucose, especially overnight. Insulin, whose main job during the day is to reduce blood glucose levels after meals, isn't produced in sufficient quantities from the pancreas.
- Type 2 diabetes has a strong genetic basis, and runs in families.
- Although over-nutrition is strongly associated with Type 2 diabetes, most people developing Type 2 aren't obese.

Type 2 diabetes is complicated and still not fully understood, but we're getting there. Until the late 1980s, we couldn't even reliably make the distinction between the two major forms of diabetes – Type 1, which usually begins in childhood and requires permanent insulin treatment right from the start, and Type 2 – but it was known that all types of diabetes were characterised by high blood glucose levels. From the late 1980s it gradually became clear that having a high glucose level wasn't the fundamental problem in Type 2. Much more important was a series of problems occurring in two organs – though these eventually led to high glucose levels.

- The liver, which in Type 2 diabetes was inefficient in processing glucose derived from absorption of food.
- The pancreas, the organ where insulin is produced. Insulin is the key hormone that reduces blood glucose levels when they rise – though, as we'll see later and in Chapter 3, insulin is amazingly versatile and has countless actions that are completely separate from its effect on blood glucose.

New ideas on the cause of Type 2 diabetes

Evidence increasingly supports the idea that most cases of Type 2 diabetes are caused by stress on the liver and pancreas resulting from over-nutrition, which usually, but not always, leads to being overweight or obese. This nutritional stress occurs over a long time – many years in some cases – before people develop diabetes. This process is similar to stress on any mechanism – for example, mechanical or even electronic equipment – where small errors and defects accumulate over the years without there being any noticeable problem, but then there is a final stress, which may not be any bigger than the earlier ones, but which precipitates mechanical or electronic failure. In the case of Type 2 diabetes, continuing stress on critical organs, the liver and pancreas, results in the onset of diabetes diagnosed by 'high' glucose levels. But the original problem will have started many years earlier, certainly in childhood, and perhaps even earlier. Around the same time as this new idea about the real nature of Type 2 diabetes was being uncovered, it was becoming clear that over-nutrition during pregnancy – and under-nutrition too – were both linked to an increased risk of Type 2 when offspring grew up to be adults. In other words, Type 2 is now considered to be a very long-term condition indeed: not caused by eating too many chocolates as a middle-aged adult, as is popularly thought, but by a series of subtle but continuing stresses that have taken place over at least a generation, and perhaps even longer.

Metabolic stress caused by over-nutrition

Let's describe in more detail the role of the liver and pancreas, how they become stressed by over-nutrition, and then how they respond to this stress.

In order to do this, and therefore to understand Type 2 diabetes, we need to appreciate that food is metabolised in a very complicated way, and we have to understand that if, for example, you eat sugar, it doesn't just go straight into the blood and register as a high glucose value. Evolution is much cleverer and more subtle than that, for the simple reason that if sugar in the diet went straight into the circulation, a blow-out on a large amount of fruit, or a box of chocolates, could raise everyone's blood glucose to dangerous levels. What occurs in the interval between eating and glucose appearing in the circulation is complicated, but it's worthwhile trying to understand it because that leads to a better understanding of the treatment of Type 2 diabetes, especially non-drug options (see Chapters 5 and 7).

> **Key point:** Overeating, but by no means always to the point of being obese, is the major cause of diabetes. Overeating stresses the function of the liver and pancreas, the two organs most involved in metabolising food.

The liver – a tough organ for tough tasks

Once food has been broken down in the intestine after eating, the products of this chemical breakdown are absorbed into the circulation and transferred to the liver for processing. If we eat a standard Western diet, most of the absorbed products (about 50–60% of the total) is glucose, which is derived from carbohydrates – primarily bread, pasta, rice and potatoes – but also 'sugar' in confectionery or sweets. This used to be sucrose, but is now mostly fructose in the form of high-fructose corn syrup and apple juice, which are ferociously sweet and found in almost every pre-prepared food. We eat smaller amounts of fats and protein, but they are also broken down into smaller chemical components and, like glucose, transferred to the liver, where they are eventually converted into glucose. Remember that not all food can be broken down, even in the chemically tough environment of the stomach and intestine. Of the non-absorbed components of food, fibre, especially soluble fibre, is highly relevant to the treatment of diabetes because it can slow down the absorption of food, and delay glucose appearing in the circulation (see Chapter 5).

The liver is the largest organ in the body, and one of the reasons it has to be so big is that it's the immediate destination of the breakdown products of all food (think about the scale of the task it faces when confronted by an all-you-can-eat buffet or 24-hour eating when its owner is on a cruise). It also processes medications, and does its best to detoxify all kinds of potentially hazardous substances we eat or even absorb from the environment. Whatever you eat – carbohydrate, fat, protein – is transported in broken-down chemical form to the liver. Once there, it's packaged up into different forms for storage. One form you're likely to remember from GCSE biology is glycogen, a starch which has been reassembled from absorbed glucose molecules. Glycogen is an efficient storage chemical but it can't be used directly to generate energy, so it has to be converted in the liver back to glucose – which is the chemical most organs need to generate energy and keep working. Both the storage of glucose as glycogen and its conversion back to glucose are performed by insulin.

High blood glucose levels first thing in the morning (that is, after fasting) are caused by an inefficient liver. Eating our daily meals causes glycogen from excess glucose to be stored in the liver. During the night when we're not eating, stored glycogen has to be chemically broken down slowly and carefully, in order to prevent our brains being starved of glucose, and to keep up with the low

Celebrating insulin

It's worthwhile pausing here to pay a brief tribute to insulin. Natural insulin is produced by the beta-cells of the pancreas; it lowers blood glucose levels by ensuring glucose is transported with great efficiency into organs that need it, mostly muscle, but to nearly every other organ as well. But insulin is also the master regulator of nearly all metabolism, and continually changes its function according to which nutrient it is dealing with (carbohydrate, some fats, or protein), which organ it's acting on, and the time of day – whether we have just finished eating or have been without food overnight. Insulin is without doubt the most versatile substance in the body, and whether naturally produced by the pancreas, or delivered from syringe or pen, deserves serious respect but not fear.

metabolic demands of the sleeping body and generally resting organs. Insulin is the key to ensuring we have just enough glucose circulating during the night, and in people without Type 2 it exerts a gentle braking effect on the liver and prevents too much glucose being released. It doesn't succeed in doing this in people with Type 2, in part because the liver becomes resistant to its effects, so there is a form of brake failure. The result is that too much glucose is released from the liver overnight, resulting in a high fasting glucose level if you measure it when you wake up.

High fasting glucose levels are very common in Type 2 diabetes, and are one of the ways in which Type 2 is diagnosed – see Chapter 2. High blood glucose levels in the morning, after what is effectively a period of overnight fasting, often puzzles people with Type 2. They are understandably at pains to point out that they don't raid the fridge in the dark hours. It isn't Type 2s who are misbehaving (unless they really do launch fridge raids); it's the liver, pancreas and your own insulin produced by the pancreas. I'll mention this again in other chapters, but if you think that diabetes is caused by eating too much sugar (sucrose, the white stuff added to hot drinks and sweets and confectionery etc.), then a high blood glucose level after eight or more hours without food doesn't stack up. This simple phenomenon tells us that Type 2 diabetes has very little to do with eating sweet sugary stuff.

Key point: People with Type 2 diabetes tend to have high blood glucose levels when they wake up. This indicates that the liver isn't working properly.

The pancreas – the insulin factory

In contrast with the liver, the pancreas is less obviously impressive, much smaller and buried at the back of the abdomen. Altogether, 90% of the pancreas produces digestive juices, while only 10% produces insulin. Insulin-producing cells, also known as beta-cells, are grouped together in 'islets'. The pancreas has important connections: it is the first stop for nutrients, especially glucose, absorbed from food in the gut. In response to these high glucose levels, in non-diabetic individuals insulin levels increase very quickly in order to lower blood glucose levels to normal.

High blood glucose levels after eating are caused by an inefficient pancreas. In people without diabetes, blood glucose levels are usually 4 or 5 mmol/l and even after eating rarely go higher than 7 or 8. If they do, they return to normal very quickly, usually within an hour. Within minutes of starting to eat (possibly even as we catch a glimpse of tempting food before we actually start eating), the pancreas is already starting to produce more insulin, which will keep blood glucose levels down. If you're eating a high-carbohydrate meal (for example, a large burger meal complete with large fries and milk shake, or lots of pasta, rice or noodles) then the healthy pancreas will go into major overdrive to produce large quantities of insulin to ensure that blood glucose levels don't rise.

It doesn't matter what form of diabetes you have; the pancreas can't produce enough insulin. In Type 1, it can't produce any at all, because the beta-cells within the islets have been destroyed by an immune process, so Type 1 people always need insulin with each meal, and even with snacks. In Type 2, there is some insulin production, but the pancreas is annoyingly sluggish and can't produce enough to cope with high carbohydrate meals. The reasons for its inefficiency are not all known, but age, degeneration of the islets and beta-cells, and – recently discovered – too much fat accumulating in the pancreas, just like too much fat in the liver (see Chapter 4), all impair the ability of this wonderful organ to produce insulin.

The result is raised blood glucose levels after meals sometimes up to 15 or 20 mmol/l, or even higher – and they don't return to pre-meal levels for perhaps four hours or longer. In many Type 2s, blood glucose levels continue to climb throughout the day, progressively higher after each carbohydrate-containing meal.

Key point: In order to keep blood glucose levels down after meals, the pancreas needs to be able to produce very large amounts of insulin.

What about fat?

We can now start putting together a picture of what's going on in Type 2 diabetes, but before doing so, I need to add one further factor that has become a major live issue in the treatment of Type 2 diabetes and its potential reversal using the stringent dietetic approach of the Newcastle team who have pioneered the approach described in Chapter 4 (see page 47). That factor is *fat*.

For the moment we'll leave aside excess belly fat (though that's important), and focus on fat stored inside the two key organs involved in Type 2: the liver and the pancreas. I will mention this again in future chapters, but excess fat, especially in the liver, is a prominent feature of pre-diabetes or the metabolic syndrome – in people whose blood glucose levels are not far off normal, but who are at very high risk of developing Type 2. We'll discuss elsewhere (see page 35) the reasons for excess fat in the liver, but in general it's caused by overloading ourselves with food – and especially carbohydrate (curiously, not fat itself, a very important fact). Excess fat in the liver, called, surprisingly clearly for the medical profession *fatty liver* (or non-alcoholic fatty liver disease), is another factor that contributes to too much glucose escaping into the circulation overnight. Fat in the liver is a good hint that we are eating too much food.

How fat are we? The Body Mass Index (BMI)

The Body Mass Index is a number that describes how overweight (or underweight) we are, allowing for our height. Your GP record will have your BMI: ask about the number if you don't already know it. If it is between 18.5 and 25, it is 'normal', 25–30 is 'overweight', over 30 is 'obese'.

You can calculate your BMI yourself if you know your weight (in kilograms) and your height (in metres).

- Multiply your height by itself (e.g. if you are 1.75 m, then 1.75 x 1.75 = 3.1). This is the 'height squared' number.
- Then take your weight (e.g. 88 kg) and *divide* it by the height squared number (e.g. 88 divided by 3.1)
- to give 28 – overweight.

Most people who develop Type 2 are overweight, but we need to get this into perspective. While the risk of developing Type 2 increases dramatically in very overweight people, at diagnosis in the UK the average BMI is right in the middle of the 'overweight' category, around 28 (as in the example above, which is my own BMI calculation). Just to remind us that, worldwide, Type 2 isn't always associated even with being overweight, the average BMI in Chinese and other people from south-east Asia is around 26 – barely overweight (see Chapter 3).

Perhaps more important than the BMI measurement of fatness is the distribution of fat, especially around the abdomen. We've discussed the critical role of excess fat stored *inside* organs, but the fat packed *around* the organs inside the abdomen is also very important in diabetes, and seems to contribute to inflammation that affects the linings of arteries, and perhaps increases the risks of heart attacks and strokes (see Chapter 11). In general, these measures of fat correlate with the amount of fat that contributes more obviously to our waist measurement, but this isn't always the case. While most people with a large tummy have excess fat inside the abdomen, there are many who don't look especially overweight but conceal a lot of this metabolically active fat inside (especially Chinese and other people from south-east Asia, and south Asians originating from India, Pakistan and Bangladesh).

Assembling the metabolic jigsaw puzzle

I've put together some of the factors we've discussed in Figure 1.1. It shows the relationships between overeating, too much fat around the abdomen, and too much fat in the liver and pancreas contributing respectively to high glucose levels first thing in the morning and high levels after meals. It's not a simple scheme, but it is important because:

- it links all the critical metabolic organs of the body
- it tells us why overeating leads to poor function of the liver and pancreas
- it explains why high blood glucose levels come at the *end* of this process – not the beginning.

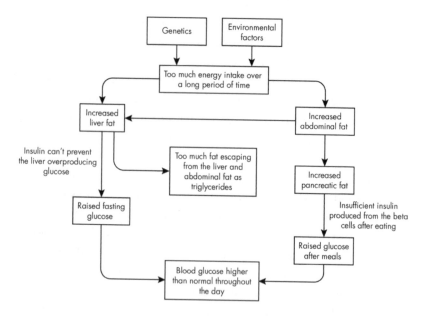

Figure 1.1: Factors contributing to Type 2 diabetes, and the relationships between these factors. Experts will argue whether one pathway is more important than the other, and the emphases may change as further evidence emerges, but this is more or less an agreed map of Type 2.

Let's discuss the two factors noted at the top of Figure 1.1: genetics and environmental causes of being overweight/obese, because they are critical to starting off the process that results in essential organs not working, and finally to high glucose levels.

Genetics – but no 'gene' therapy for the foreseeable future

Since most people developing Type 2 diabetes aren't hugely overweight, other factors must operate. Genetics is an obvious candidate, and family history plays an important part in determining the risk of developing Type 2. For example, if you have one parent with Type 2 diabetes you run a lifetime risk of around 20–30%.

That may not seem terribly high, but recall that only about 2% of the general population of the UK has Type 2 diabetes – though there are major ethnic variations which in some parts of the country give a much higher rate. If both parents are affected, the risk increases to 50%. Genetics therefore plays an important part. But if you're thinking 'What about gene therapy?' think again. There *are* unusual causes of Type 2-like diabetes caused by abnormalities in single genes that can now be easily identified on special blood tests. These are grouped together as 'Maturity Onset Diabetes of the Young' (MODY), also known as 'monogenic' diabetes, because they are caused by a single (mono) gene abnormality.

However, in the Type 2 that you have, and I might develop, researchers have found minor abnormalities in hundreds, perhaps thousands, of genes. Each contributes a tiny additional risk, and no doubt there are hundreds or thousands more yet to be discovered that will add further small risks. But I can be confident that there will never be genetic treatments for Type 2 diabetes. (The fact that countless genetic abnormalities contribute to Type 2 should make us appreciate that it is a *complicated* condition.)

Key point: Type 2 diabetes runs very strongly in families. If you have Type 2, be aware of the high risk in first-degree relatives (brothers, sisters and children). Overnutrition is the key problem.

Environmental causes – too much food or lack of exercise?

The food industry is very keen to convince us that overweight and Type 2 diabetes are not the result of eating too much of their high-appeal, high-calorie, high-sugar, high-fat products, but are caused by our not doing enough exercise. This is incorrect. The dramatic increase in diabetes seen in many countries over the past 30–40 years is mostly due to our eating more and gaining weight, and not because we are taking substantially less exercise; weight has increased more rapidly than exercise has decreased. Of course, exercise is important for heart health, can prevent weight gain after dieting has stopped and may help with certain specific diabetes complications – for example, fatty liver – but only the heaviest and most prolonged exercise regimens use sufficient energy to result in meaningful weight loss (see Chapter 8). There's no evidence that exercise prevents diabetes in susceptible people – except if you're of Chinese origin – but we've already seen that Chinese people with Type 2 diabetes are quite different from people in Westernised countries.

Summary

Overnutrition on a background of genetics is the major factor behind most cases of Type 2 diabetes. Sugars (e.g. glucose, sucrose, fructose and high-fructose corn syrup) aren't themselves the cause; in most people too much carbohydrate and fats, both high in calories, contribute to weight gain and to stressing the two organs most heavily involved in metabolising our food – the liver and pancreas. Although increasing levels of obesity are strongly associated with a higher risk of developing Type 2, in the UK most people with newly diagnosed diabetes are overweight (e.g. BMI around 28), and not obese. Certain ethnic groups, for example Chinese people, are barely overweight and yet run a high risk of diabetes.

Chapter 2

Diagnosing diabetes

Key points

- Normal blood glucose levels rarely go above 4–6 mmol/l, except for a short time after a meal.
- Diabetes is diagnosed when fasting glucose levels are 7.0 mmol/l or above, or more than 11.1 when there are obvious symptoms of high glucose – for example, excessive thirst or weight loss.
- Most people don't have symptoms when they are diagnosed on a blood test.
- In many people, high glucose levels have been present but undetected for years before diagnosis.
- Occasionally, diabetes presents with a serious complication, such as a heart attack or stroke.

Chapter 1 described an up-to-date view of the origins of diabetes, and we saw that Type 2 is caused by a combination of a strong genetic susceptibility to diabetes and overnutrition that stresses the liver and pancreas, which then no longer work together in harmony to maintain stable low blood glucose levels. Dysfunctional insulin produced by the pancreas leads to glucose escaping from the liver overnight, and to blood glucose levels remaining high after a carbohydrate-rich meal. Abnormal insulin also leads to high blood pressure and abnormal cholesterol balance, and to a host of other important problems that are often overlooked while we focus too much on blood glucose levels (these problems are covered in Chapter 3). However, we can't get away from the fact that although Type 2 diabetes is much, much more than 'just' a high blood glucose level, diagnosing it has always been based on the precise measurement of blood glucose.

Blood glucose tests in context

It's worthwhile knowing a little about the history of *why* blood glucose has been the standard way to diagnose diabetes, and will remain so. As we saw in Chapter 1, it's only over the past 30 years or so that we have been able to make a reliable distinction between Type 1 and Type 2 diabetes.

In Type 1 diabetes, the kind of diabetes that usually affects children and adolescents, the condition develops suddenly and the only organ to misbehave is the pancreas, where insulin is produced; therefore in this type of diabetes *the only problem* appeared to be high blood glucose levels. High blood pressure and blood vessel disorders – for example, in the heart and kidneys – certainly occur after many years with Type 1, but until recently they were still thought to be caused by persisting high glucose levels resulting from imperfect insulin treatment (since the pancreas fails almost completely in Type 1 diabetes, insulin is needed immediately and permanently). So it's easy to understand why diabetes starting later in life was considered to be more or less the same condition as Type 1, though usually with a less scary onset. (The distinction was further blurred by the fact that between 1921 when insulin was first used in humans and the 1950s, the only treatments for any type of diabetes were diet and insulin.)

At this early stage of research into diabetes, epidemiologists (scientists who study disease in populations rather than individuals) measured blood glucose levels in large numbers of people so they could establish a 'number' that could be used to diagnose diabetes. They focused exclusively on blood glucose levels, and did not take account of, for example, blood pressure and lipids such as HDL cholesterol and triglycerides that we now know are as important as blood glucose in determining the long-term outcomes of Type 2. But since all diabetes at the time was considered to be a condition of high blood glucose levels, and because blood glucose can be measured reliably, easily and cheaply, that's what they focused on. The unintended result of all this blood glucose-measuring activity is that Type 2 diabetes is still considered by many professionals and patients to be predominantly a problem of high blood glucose levels. Nevertheless, we have to accept that blood glucose will remain *the* diagnostic test for Type 2 diabetes, and we therefore need to understand the numbers that have been agreed, while always bearing in mind that high glucose is only the easily measurable tip of a large iceberg of other problems.

> **Key point:** Although Type 2 diabetes usually includes high blood pressure and abnormal cholesterol levels as well as high blood glucose levels, historically we've always used blood glucose values to diagnose it.

What are 'normal' blood glucose levels?

Before discussing the blood glucose levels we use to diagnose diabetes, we need to get an idea of what are normal glucose levels in people who don't have diabetes. We'll defer the prickly problem of 'pre-diabetes' (the grey zone between strictly normal blood glucose levels and definite diabetes) until Chapter 3.

Figure 2.1 shows glucose levels monitored continuously over 24 hours in a thin young person – that is, someone at zero risk of having undiagnosed diabetes. Clock time runs along the bottom, from midnight to midnight. The test was run over four days, so there are four different lines (the average measurement is shown with a dotted line).

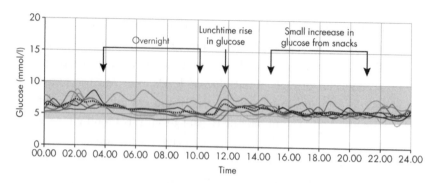

Figure 2.1: Glucose measurements taken continuously in a young, non-diabetic person of normal weight over four consecutive days.

I always find tracings like Figure 2.1 remarkable: glucose levels nearly always lie between 4 and 6 mmol/l. As you might expect, the graph looks even flatter and lower during the night (on the left), while during the day there are small blips caused by eating, especially around midday, when the subject seems to have eaten her highest-carbohydrate meal of the day. One day, the lunchtime blip is higher, reaching nearly 10 mmol/l. (This is an important point for Type 2s. Many would be disturbed to find a peak blood glucose of 10 shortly after a meal, but you can see that this is common in people without diabetes; the key point is how quickly the values return to normal – within about an hour in a non-diabetic individual, but up to three or even five hours in someone with Type 2.) Because blood glucose levels rise briefly after meals even in non-diabetic individuals, fasting glucose levels (eight hours or more after food) are used for diagnosis, as they are at their lowest and most stable in the fasting state.

Key point: In someone without diabetes, blood glucose levels are usually in the range 4–6 mmol/l, though they can rise to 10 or even perhaps higher for a very short time after a large meal, particularly if it contained lots of carbohydrates.

Another (very important) **key point:** Although non-diabetic glucose levels are usually 4–6 mmol/l, there is no advantage (and possibly some harm) in aiming for these low levels if you have diabetes, especially if you are taking insulin. In general, values between 6 and 10 mmol/l are near-ideal for all people taking medication or insulin (or both).

The time frame over which Type 2 diabetes develops

Type 1 diabetes develops very rapidly, usually over a few weeks, because the pancreas fails suddenly and permanently. The young people affected usually lose weight dramatically, often have raging thirst and can pass urine every few minutes, and feel weak and dreadful. This is what happens when blood glucose levels suddenly surge and stay there for a few weeks – most people with newly diagnosed Type 1 have glucose levels of 20 mmol/l or higher. This dramatic onset of symptoms is unusual in Type 2 diabetes, where the process is played out over a much longer time frame – years rather than weeks. However, we'll see that this still occurs in Type 2 when the blood glucose levels rise sufficiently high and stay there.

The characteristic slow progression of Type 2, which causes no symptoms for a long time, was documented in what is called the 'Whitehall study' of British civil servants (see Reference section page 209). Blood glucose levels were measured every year until the expected small proportion of them developed diabetes (see Figure 2.2). Over the course of 10 years, the average fasting glucose levels rose only slightly, from 5.5 to 5.8 mmol/l, but a year before diagnosis it increased from 5.8 to 6.3, and then to 7.0 (which, as we will see, is the level at which Type 2 is diagnosed). The slow rise in the previous 10 years explains why an occasional blood glucose taken over this period will usually be normal, while the rapid rise in the two years preceding diagnosis explains why some people with Type 2 can have symptoms of high blood glucose for several months before diagnosis. The slow-then-fast trajectory accounts for the different ways Type 2 is diagnosed, and that's what we will discuss next.

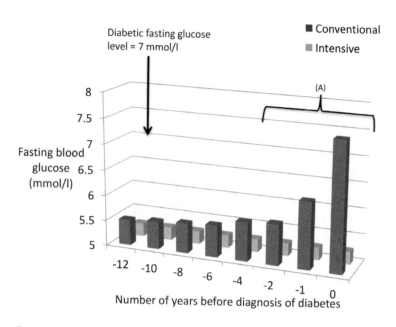

Figure 2.2: Blood glucose levels in the Whitehall study of civil servants. In people who go on to develop Type 2 diabetes, blood glucose levels rise very slowly for many years until about two years before diagnosis, when they increase from just under 6 mmol/l to 7 (A). Although this is the diagnostic value for diabetes, nobody has symptoms at this level. Follow-up stopped at this point, but you can see that if blood glucose levels continue to rise at the same fast rate, many people will start developing symptoms over the next year or two when they reach 12–13 or higher – this happens frequently in real life, in contrast to research studies where blood glucose levels are measured every year.

Diabetes diagnosed on a blood test without any symptoms of diabetes

These days most people are unaware they have diabetes until they have a routine blood test requested for other reasons (for example, many people with high blood pressure have a blood glucose test with their annual tests of kidney and liver function; a good idea, as hypertension is itself a risk factor for developing Type 2). Increasingly, people are self-diagnosing by doing a finger-prick blood glucose test using someone else's meter. There's one practical point: a high blood glucose won't come up on a routine blood test because glucose needs a separate sample taken into a different blood tube, usually colour-coded yellow. If you're concerned about your risk of developing Type 2, ask specifically for a blood glucose test.

What blood glucose level defines diabetes?

We now have to grasp the nettle, and mention the values needed to diagnose Type 2 diabetes. Amazingly, the whole world agrees that a *fasting* glucose level of 7.0 mmol/l or above is the diagnostic level. (It used to be 7.8, but relatively recently it has been revised downwards and it is unlikely to change again.) The reason the world agreed on 7.0 and above is that complications specifically due to diabetes – for example, those involving the retina of the eye (see Chapter 11) – almost never occur in people with values under 7.0.

> **Key point:** Diabetes is diagnosed when a fasting glucose level is 7.0 mmol/l or higher. This measurement needs to be made in a laboratory – finger-prick blood tests using home glucose meters may give a broad indication, but aren't accurate enough to make such an important diagnosis.

We can make an interesting observation from the non-diabetic glucose tracing in Figure 2.1. Glucose in a non-diabetic person runs between 4 and 6 mmol/l, yet diabetes is diagnosed when the value is only apparently slightly higher – that is, 7 or above. So it's no surprise that most people diagnosed with diabetes have no symptoms.

The HbA₁c test for diagnosis of Type 2

More recently most, but in this case not all, of the world has agreed that a specialised blood test known as the glycated haemoglobin (HbA_{1c}) test can be used to diagnose diabetes. HbA_{1c} indicates how high average blood glucose levels have been over the previous six to eight weeks. All people with diabetes are familiar with HbA_{1c}, which has been used from the early 1980s to *monitor* diabetes annually or more frequently. We are less familiar using the test to diagnose diabetes, but you can see why it might be helpful. It could indicate whether someone has intermittently slightly high blood glucose measurements that wouldn't be apparent on an occasional blood glucose test, and it would be particularly valuable in those Type 2s who have almost normal fasting glucose levels but who develop high values after meals. Because it looks backwards at the general blood glucose level, HbA_{1c} gives the same result whatever time of day it's measured, so unlike a diagnostic blood glucose test, it doesn't have to be taken when fasting. HbA_{1c}, like glucose, requires a separate blood tube, so it won't be measured on a 'routine' blood test, and the result will take a few days to come back, compared with the glucose level which will return within a day (even quicker if the laboratory finds it is very high). HbA_{1c} isn't accepted worldwide as a test for diabetes, but it's still useful.

The accuracy of blood glucose and HbA_{1c} measurements made the 'oral glucose tolerance test' obsolete, except in pregnancy. The aim of this test was to measure how well the body coped with a large (very large) dose of glucose. Blood glucose tests were taken fasting and two hours after the glucose drink. Although this test should have hit the history books about 10 years ago, it still surfaces occasionally, as it is still available in hospitals for diagnosing diabetes during pregnancy.

> **Key point:** An HbA$_{1c}$ of 6.5% or more (45 mmol/mol in the units introduced in 2011) can be used to diagnose diabetes.

Symptoms of diabetes caused by high blood glucose levels

Urinary symptoms

In non-diabetic people, the body has a remarkable ability to hang on to glucose. This shouldn't be a surprise: when humans didn't have access to regular food, which was the case for nearly all of us until very recently, it was imperative to retain as much glucose as possible so that the body – and especially the brain – could continue functioning. This responsibility for preciously guarding glucose fell to the kidneys: they filter thousands of litres of blood every day. Kidneys have a very effective mechanism for reabsorbing glucose from the urine back into the circulation. The result is that people without diabetes (and many with well-controlled diabetes) almost never have detectable glucose in the urine.

However, when blood glucose levels rise above about 10 mmol/l, the kidney's glucose-retaining mechanism finds it difficult to cope, and glucose starts leaking into the urine. The higher the blood glucose level, the more finds its way into the urine. This has several consequences. First, when glucose passes into the urine, it takes extra salt and water along with it. The result: excessive urine, so that sometimes people with high blood glucose levels end up peeing very frequently, day and night. Excessive loss of glucose, salt and water in the urine leads to thirst, and many people start drinking water during the night as well as visiting the loo, and carrying large bottles of water around with them. Second, because glucose is the body's major source of energy, if it is lost in the urine then it isn't available to be used by the muscles. Result: unintentional weight loss. At first, losing some weight is often welcomed, but if it continues, it's clear something's not right.

Throughout this book I'm doing my best not to focus on specific drug treatments, as I think they get quite sufficient publicity, but it's worth noting that scientists have exploited this kidney mechanism to develop a new class of diabetes drugs. These are the 'flozin' drugs, also called 'SGLT2 inhibitors' – for example, dapagliflozin, canagliflozin and empagliflozin. They prevent the kidney reabsorbing glucose from the urine, so deliberately encourage loss of glucose – in a gentle and controlled way, of course. More urinary glucose means lower blood glucose levels, and with the energy lost, some weight reduction. The downside is that some people tend to pee excessively when they take these newer medications, and there is a risk of the fungal infection thrush.

Infections and blurred vision

Like humans, bugs (bacteria and fungi) love glucose and thrive on it. So, genital irritation due to thrush (the candida fungus) is common when glucose levels are high. Also, although not so common these days, bacterial skin infections, such as boils, can occur when blood glucose levels have been high for a long time. Finally, if glucose levels remain high for weeks, the lens of the eye becomes dehydrated, and intermittent blurred vision is a well-known symptom. It often prompts a visit to the optometrist, who is likely to recognise the symptom and confirm it with an eye examination. (Because this symptom takes a long time to develop, blurred vision doesn't settle until a few weeks after blood glucose levels fall.)

Many people developing these reversible symptoms of diabetes have blood glucose levels in the range 15–20 mmol/l. The rules allow a diagnosis of Type 2 diabetes if someone has these symptoms and a blood glucose level measured at any time of day, not necessarily fasting, is 11.1 mmol/l or higher. Because the diagnosis of diabetes has significant consequences for people and their families, a repeat test – after fasting – is sometimes needed, but if the blood test was done in a laboratory and is very high, then there's no need for a repeat (an HbA_{1c} measurement would confirm the diabetes, and give an indication of how high the average blood glucose had been over the past few weeks).

Symptoms of the complications of diabetes

Most people, like the civil servants in the Whitehall study mentioned earlier, slide very gently into diabetes. But there is another, fortunately much smaller, group who seem to have had glucose levels well into the diabetes range for years before they are diagnosed. I have encountered several people who clearly describe periods where they have had symptoms of diabetes that have then settled, perhaps of their own accord, or with weight loss or increased exercise, only for the symptoms to return and then to have the diagnosis confirmed. They often have detectable diabetes complications affecting the blood vessels, and sometimes symptoms of nerve damage in the feet – for example, numbness, or pins and needles, and in men often accompanied by erectile dysfunction. Using information on the most specific of these complications (retinopathy affecting the eye), the epidemiologists calculate that diabetic blood glucose levels have been present for an average of seven years, but we will see in Chapter 3 that other factors that stress the blood vessels tend to cluster with high glucose levels – the metabolic syndrome. So over the seven years that blood glucose levels were high, there is likely to be high blood pressure, abnormal cholesterol levels and an increased tendency for the blood to clot. All these are likely to have gone undetected (and may have been made worse by smoking), and it's not surprising that some people are first diagnosed with diabetes when they are admitted to hospital with one of its most serious complications – a heart attack.

In the early 2000s it was found that up to one third of patients admitted to hospital with a heart attack had diabetes that had not been diagnosed before their admission. This still occurs frequently: a double and terrible shock – newly diagnosed diabetes *and* a heart attack. The first inkling some patients have of their diabetes is a stroke or mini-stroke (transient ischaemic attack or TIA).

This highlights two themes we'll discuss further: first, mild but persistent elevations in blood glucose levels that do not cause symptoms, but nevertheless contribute to the long-term complications of diabetes. The sudden rise around the time of diagnosis (or, indeed, after an occasional blow-out meal) comes as a shock, but except in very rare cases does not cause serious problems. Second, Type 2 diabetes can cause undetected damage to blood vessels throughout the body. This leads to the question, still unresolved, whether people at risk of diabetes should be screened every so often. The discussion would occupy books much larger than this one, but there are simple questionnaires that can indicate your risk of diabetes – for example, the one promoted by Diabetes UK. If you are at risk, don't forget to nudge other members of your family to estimate their risk, as Type 2 runs so strongly within families.

Summary

Although Type 2 diabetes is not just a condition of high blood glucose levels, measuring glucose goes back a long way and is cheap and reliable. Diabetes is diagnosed when fasting glucose levels are 7.0 mmol/l or higher, compared with 4–6 in people without diabetes. Most people don't have symptoms at blood glucose levels of 7–10 (and these may have been present undetected and without symptoms for many years), but higher values result in glucose leaking into the urine, causing thirst, frequent toilet visits and occasionally weight loss, blurred vision and an increased risk of fungal and bacterial infections. A few people first find out about their Type 2 diabetes when they have a major illness, usually involving blockages to blood vessels, especially heart attacks and strokes.

Chapter 3

Pre-diabetes and the metabolic syndrome

Key points

- Pre-diabetes, like diabetes itself, is defined using fasting blood glucose levels – somewhere between 'normal' and diabetes (6.1–6.9 mmol/l).
- Most research has concentrated on reducing the risk of people with pre-diabetes progressing to diabetes (that is blood glucose levels of 7.0 or higher).
- Pre-diabetes is more than just a glucose number, and is often associated with being overweight or obese, high blood pressure and unbalanced cholesterol levels. When it clusters like this it is called the metabolic syndrome, or the insulin resistance syndrome.
- Other medical conditions associated with the metabolic syndrome include polycystic ovary syndrome, gout, obstructive sleep apnoea and even – speculatively – Alzheimer's disease.
- The factor linking these very different conditions is insulin itself. Although insulin is important in keeping blood glucose levels under control, it has multiple actions in several organs that are separate from its role in regulating blood glucose.

Grey areas always generate big arguments

As we saw in Chapter 2, non-diabetic blood glucose levels run between 4 and 6 mmol/l (with occasional brief excursions to 8–10 immediately after big carbohydrate-containing meals). Diabetes is diagnosed once fasting blood glucose levels rise above 7 mmol/l. So what about blood glucose levels that lie slightly higher than 'normal' but lower than the level used to diagnose diabetes? Can glucose levels in this grey area affect health?

Grey areas in everything are often major battle grounds, and there's no difference here. Academics fall out with each other, while major international organisations have more measured 'disagreements'. The difficulty is understanding where 'normality' ends and the grey zone starts. For example, the American Diabetes Association considers any blood glucose level of more than 5.5 mmol/l to be higher than normal, while the rest of the world uses a threshold of 6.1.

The problem is that there are so many people with fasting levels of 5.5. mmol/l or just higher that if we used this number to define even mild abnormality, then probably one-third of the world's population would be included. Currently, in most countries, fasting glucose measurements between 6.1 and 6.9 mmol/l are considered slightly high, though not quite diabetes. But is all this numerical nit-picking of any real importance to people?

Key point: Pre-diabetes is associated with a fasting glucose level of between 6.1 and 6.9 mmol/l. It indicates an increased risk of developing diabetes and therefore its complications, but by itself it should be considered a gentle warning of future trouble, and not itself a 'disease' that needs 'treatment'.

Broadly speaking, the situation in pre-diabetes is the same as the one we see in confirmed diabetes. Diabetes was originally defined as a fasting blood glucose level (7.0 mmol/l), above which people can develop complications that only occur in diabetes. The easiest of these to detect is diabetic eye disease (retinopathy; see Chapter 11). So, although we define diabetes using a blood glucose level (7.0 mmol/l or higher), that number is much less important to the individual than the risk of developing complications of diabetes. Similarly, with pre-diabetes. Discussion about whether 5.5 or 6.1 is 'abnormal' is much less important than whether there are any associated medical problems with any values in the grey zone. There are, as we'll discuss shortly. First, though, let's look at the risk of developing definite diabetes, defined as a fasting glucose level of 7.0 or higher, if you have pre-diabetes.

Pre-diabetes and the risk of developing full-blown diabetes

If you have pre-diabetic blood glucose levels, can you do anything to postpone a further rise into the diabetes range? There are a number of studies that have investigated reducing the risk of progressing from pre-diabetes to diabetes and which included large numbers of individuals studied over several years. We can now benefit from the long-term results of these trials, which started in the 1980s and continued into the early 2000s. Because pre-diabetes is not a 'disease' or 'illness' itself, most of the trials used lifestyle intervention (weight loss and exercise), though there were also a few drug-based studies.

Broadly speaking – and there's no surprise here – the trials confirm that consistent weight loss, though not always a spectacular amount, and regular exercise do indeed delay progression to diabetic blood glucose levels. Most studies combined a portfolio of both weight loss and increased exercise, so it's not possible to separate out whether one intervention was more effective than the other. However, in a study in Chinese people (the Da Qing study – see References for this chapter, page 211) one group was given an exercise schedule (the aim was to increase daily activity by 10–30 minutes, depending on the intensity of exercise), the other encouraged to lose weight (actual weight loss was 1.5–2.5 kg). All interventions reduced the risk of progressing to Type 2 by between

30 and 45% – diet, exercise and exercise plus diet were about equally effective. We should be cautious in extending conclusions from this population (average BMI was only slightly overweight, 26) to a more overweight population, especially when it comes to recommending increased exercise as a way of reducing progression from pre-diabetes.

> **Key point:** Consistent weight loss and increased activity levels significantly reduce the risk of progressing from pre-diabetes to diabetes. In Chinese people increased exercise alone was effective.

Can medication postpone the onset of diabetes?

One study, the Diabetes Prevention Program in the USA (see references on page 210), found that in younger people (those aged 35–40), and those who were particularly overweight, metformin – as used in the treatment of Type 2 diabetes itself – helped, to a certain extent, to reduce the likelihood of developing diabetes. However, metformin was considerably less effective than the lifestyle portfolio (6 kg weight loss over four years and increased exercise up to 150 minutes/week), and the effect only persisted while people were taking medication. After stopping the tablets, blood glucose levels went up immediately, whereas blood glucose levels remained lower in people who had been in the lifestyle group. Although weight (and therefore blood glucose) often increases after you've stopped dieting, it doesn't do so suddenly.

> **Key point:** Medication (metformin) is less effective than lifestyle in preventing the onset of Type 2 diabetes, and its effect lasts only as long as the medication is taken.

Does pre-diabetes have health consequences?

Because pre-diabetes is diagnosed using blood glucose levels, I've already mentioned there's a risk we'll become obsessed with minute differences in numbers. If you have a blood glucose level that's in the lower pre-diabetes range, say 6.2 mmol/l, is that 'better' than one that's nearly at the diabetes level, for example 6.8? If it's lower, then you are probably farther away from developing a diabetic blood glucose level of 7, but that may not be of great importance. People remain in the pre-diabetic range for a long time, perhaps nearly the whole of their adult lifetime. So, if we're only going to get concerned once blood glucose levels increase from 6.7 to 7.0, then we may be missing major health concerns if pre-diabetes persists for a long time. And yes, there are significant health problems that are associated with pre-diabetes. The important thing is not to regard it just as a 'borderline' glucose level that needs an occasional follow-up blood test. In a world obsessed with numbers and targets, this is a risk that shows no sign of going away. We should be more concerned with health outcomes that matter to people.

The clinical triallists of the 1990s and 2000s looked in a limited way at the long-term health consequences of pre-diabetes. Because the studies initially focused on blood glucose levels, the possible broader associations of pre-diabetes, especially cardiac disease, weren't studied, so long-term blood glucose outcomes continued to be reported. In general, people who had successfully achieved weight loss and exercise goals during the trials (which usually lasted three to five years) were at lower risk of developing Type 2 when followed up for several more years. But that's not an earth-shattering finding, as people who had done well initially with exercise and weight loss were the most likely to continue.

However, the long-term outcomes of the Chinese Da Qing study mentioned above (and see References on page 211) were truly unexpected: 20 years after the end of the trial, those who had initially done well with exercise or weight loss had a 40% lower risk of heart disease. Of course, the risk of blood glucose climbing into the diabetes range was reduced as well – by about 50%. From other studies, though, it doesn't look as if Europeans and Americans benefit quite as much. Nevertheless, a study in Finland found that pre-diabetic people who initially managed to maintain their lower weight and better diet continued to do so, as well as having a lower risk of crossing the blood glucose threshold into diabetes.

Key point: Although exercise and weight loss reduce the risk of developing diabetic blood glucose levels, they don't reduce the risk of developing serious diabetes outcomes such as heart disease – except in Chinese individuals. We don't know the reasons for these ethnic differences.

The metabolic syndrome

Let's try and think more broadly than blood glucose. If you have pre-diabetic blood glucose levels, then you are more likely to have certain other conditions associated with it. A recognised combination of conditions or features is called a 'syndrome'. This combination has been given various names, including 'syndrome X' (the original title), the 'insulin resistance syndrome' and, probably the most descriptive term and the one we'll use here, the 'metabolic syndrome'. Because they are all associated with mildly abnormal blood glucose levels, people diagnosed with Type 2 diabetes usually have features of the metabolic syndrome, but there are also many people with strictly non-diabetic glucose levels who also have the metabolic syndrome.

Figure 3.1 shows the widespread impact of the metabolic syndrome on different parts of the body. Some of these associations are not obvious (acne and gout, for example), and certainly not clearly linked with higher glucose levels.

The link is thought to lie in the many roles played by insulin – completely separate from its best-known job of reducing blood glucose levels. It's not surprising that over millions of years insulin has developed lots of different jobs, because – after all – it is the master regulator of the body's metabolism. We mentioned this much wider and very interesting spectrum in Chapter 1. Even when blood glucose is at levels that everyone can agree are normal, abnormal insulin action poses some major health hazards years, perhaps decades, before blood glucose levels become 'high' – another reason not to fixate on minute differences in nearly normal glucose values.

Key point: The health consequences of the metabolic syndrome are due to insulin acting in abnormal ways that are not linked to its effect on blood glucose.

As with diabetes, the metabolic syndrome was (and still is) formally defined using simple measurements:
- Obesity (high waist circumference – for example, more than 40 inches in men or 35 inches in women. No cheating when you're measuring it – as if. The measurement must be taken at the level of the belly button, not the hips.
- Intermediate – pre-diabetic – glucose levels (6.1 to 6.9 mmol/l).
- High blood pressure (systolic pressure more than 140 mm).
- Relatively normal cholesterol levels, but other lipid (fat) values are abnormal – for example, low protective HDL cholesterol levels, and higher triglyceride levels.

The scientific definition requires obesity together with one of the others to be present, but in real life we need to be much more flexible, because any, all or none of these might warrant treatment in an individual. I'll discuss some of the features of the definition

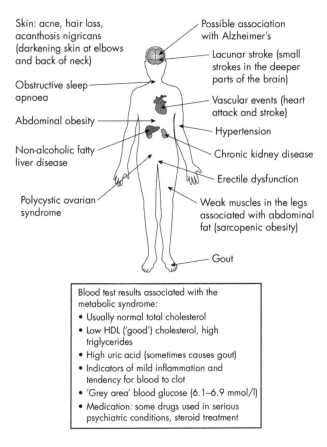

Skin: acne, hair loss, acanthosis nigricans (darkening skin at elbows and back of neck)

Obstructive sleep apnoea

Abdominal obesity

Non-alcoholic fatty liver disease

Polycystic ovarian syndrome

Possible association with Alzheimer's

Lacunar stroke (small strokes in the deeper parts of the brain)

Vascular events (heart attack and stroke)

Hypertension

Chronic kidney disease

Erectile dysfunction

Weak muscles in the legs associated with abdominal fat (sarcopenic obesity)

Gout

Blood test results associated with the metabolic syndrome:
- Usually normal total cholesterol
- Low HDL ('good') cholesterol, high triglycerides
- High uric acid (sometimes causes gout)
- Indicators of mild inflammation and tendency for blood to clot
- 'Grey area' blood glucose (6.1–6.9 mmol/l)
- Medication: some drugs used in serious psychiatric conditions, steroid treatment

Figure 3.1: Some features of the metabolic syndrome.

itself, and then go on to discuss other and less obvious clinical associations.

Hypertension (high blood pressure)

High blood pressure is very strongly linked with both pre-diabetes and Type 2 (see Chapter 10). Embarrassingly, and in spite of decades of research, the link is mostly unexplained, but the odds are on insulin causing salt retention, one of the key features of hypertension. A good follow-on question from this would be: do hypertensive people who don't have Type 2 have features of the metabolic syndrome? Answer: yes, many of them do. The general message is that in individuals with any features of the metabolic syndrome, we should look around for the other commonly associated features.

As discussed in more detail in Chapter 10, blood pressure is recorded using two numbers. The first ('upper') number, known as the 'systolic' blood pressure, is the only relevant one, as it reflects the peak blood pressure exerted on the major blood vessels during contraction of the heart and is therefore the measurement most strongly related to arterial damage. The definition of hypertension in the metabolic syndrome is the same as the one we use generally: systolic pressure consistently 140 mm Hg or higher.

> **Key point:** Hypertension is a common feature of the metabolic syndrome.

Abnormal blood lipid (fat) profile

The formal metabolic syndrome definition also includes a characteristic combination, easily detected by a blood test (and often measured at the same time as total cholesterol): a low level of protective ('good') HDL cholesterol, which contributes to heart disease and stroke risk, and high triglyceride levels, which are more associated with food excess, especially carbohydrates. The formal definitions are triglycerides higher than 1.7 mmol/l, and HDL cholesterol lower than 1.0 mmol/l in men, and 1.2 in women. Insulin's involvement here? Probably in the biochemical pathways in the cell where one form of fat (lipid) is converted to another. It's worthwhile noting again that these processes have nothing to do with glucose metabolism or blood glucose levels.

Fatty liver: too much fat in the liver (and in other organs)

If you have an ultrasound scan of the abdomen for any reason, the technician or radiologist will often take at least a quick look at the liver; excess fat there is a common finding, regardless of the reason for the initial ultrasound request. 'Fatty liver' is the usual term, but because excess alcohol is a common cause of fat in the liver, when it isn't a contributor (that is, alcohol intake is less than the recommended level, currently 14 units a week), it's called 'non-alcoholic fatty liver disease', usually abbreviated to 'NAFLD'. Fatty liver is rather like high blood pressure. Perhaps 30 to 40% of people with no whiff of diabetes according to glucose levels are hypertensive, but once they've progressed to Type 2, 80–90% have high blood pressure. The same goes for fatty liver: it's very common in non-diabetic people, but affects about three-quarters of Type 2s.

Fatty liver/NAFLD isn't usually considered one of the classical 'complications' of diabetes, which mostly affect small blood vessels and large arteries (see Chapter 11), but alarm bells about long-term (chronic) liver disease developing from fatty liver have been ringing increasingly loudly over the past few years. It starts, as we'll see, with a metabolic abnormality – that is, insulin not doing what it should, this time in relation to fats which are manufactured in the liver. But fat that has been in liver cells for several years can set up a low level of inflammation – a non-infectious form of hepatitis. In most people the inflammation remains unchanged during their lifetime, but, for unknown reasons, in a small number the irritant effect of the inflammation stimulates the liver to try to seal off the inflammation with tough fibrous tissue. After decades, the result can be cirrhosis where all the functions of the liver – and there are lots – fail. Although only a very small proportion of people with Type 2 will progress in this way, there is concern because Type 2 is very common and large total numbers of people might be affected.

> **Key point:** Fatty liver is detectable on ultrasound scan in many overweight people who have neither diabetic nor pre-diabetic blood glucose levels.

What causes fatty liver?

It's worth pausing to discuss this, because it not only expands our awareness of the complications of Type 2 diabetes and pre-diabetes, but also adds to our understanding of the range of insulin's functions that are not related to glucose levels. In fact, insulin behaves here in a similar way to how it does with glucose. You'll remember from Chapter 1 how, in diabetic people, the liver leaks too much glucose (especially overnight) as a result of insulin not working well enough. What should be a gentle drip of the glucose tap turns into quite a big trickle. In fatty liver, though, we need to substitute a fat – triglycerides – for the glucose.

Triglycerides are synthesised from the carbohydrates we eat, and are stored (like glycogen) in the liver. Fructose, mostly now found as high-fructose corn syrup, and used as a sweetener in a huge number of manufactured products, especially non-diet soft drinks, is thought to be a particularly powerful factor in producing triglycerides. The liver itself also produces triglycerides. In people without diabetes, insulin keeps triglycerides neatly tucked away in the liver, except for very small amounts that get into the circulation from where they are used as a fuel, like glucose, to produce energy, though triglycerides do so less efficiently than glucose. In the metabolic syndrome and Type 2, insulin is less effective at preventing the liver making triglycerides, and, as in the situation with glucose, less effective at keeping it there. The liver becomes overloaded with triglycerides and related molecules, and that's effectively the recipe for producing fatty liver.

We see this picture at its most dramatic when people with insulin-treated diabetes (usually Type 1, but also in Type 2) stop taking their insulin for whatever reason. As well as glucose leaking from the liver in large quantities, so do triglycerides. When this happens, people usually need hospital treatment for very high glucose levels, but triglycerides can be sky-high too – sometimes values of 50–100 mmol/l, compared with the usual levels of 2 mmol/l or less. It's easy to spot: blood taken from a vein for a routine test looks creamy pink, sometimes barely red at all, because it contains so much fat. In some cases, the inflammatory effect of the high blood triglyceride level can cause pancreatitis, a severe and dangerous inflammation of the pancreas (see Figure 3.2).

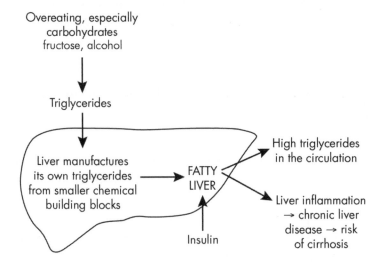

Figure 3.2: Fatty liver. Triglycerides produced both from food and by the liver itself pack the liver cells. In pre-diabetes and Type 2 diabetes insulin is less effective at ensuring triglycerides do not escape from the liver into the circulation. Fatty liver and high blood triglyceride levels are common in the metabolic syndrome.

Treating fatty liver

Dramatic weight loss is the best way of reducing fat in the liver (see Chapter 4). There is optimism that bariatric surgery may be of benefit even when fatty liver disease is fairly advanced.

Interestingly, high levels of physical training (for example 30–40 minutes a week for 12 weeks) reduces the amount of fat in the liver, even if there isn't weight loss (see Chapter 8). It looks as if exercise has quite a specific effect here. There have also been several trials of drugs, many of them blood-glucose lowering drugs used in established Type 2; however, despite great hopes, none has shown improvement in the structure of the liver, which is what matters.

Key point: Exercise and weight loss are the most effective treatments for fatty liver. No drug treatment is conclusively effective.

Fat in other organs: an emerging area of interest in pre-diabetes

Although fat in the liver is easy to detect and very common, excess fat can accumulate in other organs, probably also through a combination of excess food and ineffective insulin. We'll see in Chapter 4 that excess fat in the pancreas is now thought to be conspiring with fatty liver to account for the metabolic problems seen in Type 2 diabetes, and that substantial weight loss can dramatically reduce fat in both these key organs, with rapidly beneficial effects on blood glucose levels and the action of insulin. If fat in the liver and pancreas can have such profound metabolic effects, then can fat in other organs also have health consequences? This is a new area of research, but interest is growing. For example, excess fat around the heart can get very close to coronary arteries, and inflammation in this fat may be responsible for thickening of the coronary arteries and contribute to heart attack risk. Normal kidneys are surrounded by a substantial cushion of fat, which may not just be there to protect against trauma. Inflammation in this fat may worsen hypertension and increase protein leakage into the urine (see Chapter 11). We'll also see in Chapter 12 that when excess fat accumulates in muscle, especially the legs, it can contribute to weakness, unsteadiness, falls and frailty in the elderly.

'Type 3' diabetes and a link with Alzheimer's?

In the past few years, metabolic syndrome characteristics have been linked to a higher risk of developing Alzheimer's disease. Research is in the very early stages and there is understandably great interest in this whole new area. There has been no shortage of dramatic headlines, to the point where 'diabetes of the brain' has been – prematurely – dubbed 'Type 3' diabetes. The brain is one of the few organs where insulin *isn't* required for glucose uptake – glucose in the circulation goes straight into brain tissue so it can prioritise supplying the energy demands of billions of nerve cells, regardless of what is happening elsewhere in the body. Nevertheless, insulin is needed in the brain for a wide variety of chemical pathways, many of them involved in lipids similar to cholesterol which are needed to maintain the structure of brain cells. In other words, this is yet another example of insulin being critical to life, though definitely not through its effects on glucose. The ultimate question is whether controlling the metabolic syndrome will result in a lower risk of dementia in older age. I have no doubt that trials will be done, but the results are a good way off just yet. However, it reminds us again that the metabolic syndrome, whether or not it progresses to Type 2 diabetes diagnosed with a high glucose level, may have long-term effects on several aspects of health – some quite unexpected.

Polycystic ovary syndrome (PCOS)

Polycystic ovary syndrome is one of the conditions associated with the metabolic syndrome that is quite well understood, and abnormal insulin is clearly the culprit here. Affected women have infrequent menstrual cycles (periods) – sometimes as few as two a year – and in severe cases some degree of infertility. Cosmetically it can be very troublesome as well, as it is frequently associated with severe acne, hirsutism (excess hair on the face and body), and hair fall from the head. Many women with PCOS are overweight, but some can be very slim. Insulin action at the ovary is the problem here. It's particularly interesting because PCOS often responds to treatment with the diabetes drug metformin, and sometimes this simple treatment restores periods and even fertility. In this instance, metformin isn't being used to reduce blood glucose levels as it is in usual cases of Type 2, but to improve the efficiency of insulin action.

> **Key point:** Polycystic ovary syndrome is caused by abnormal insulin action, but is frequently seen in normal-weight women who have normal glucose levels.

Finally, let's briefly consider two conditions undoubtedly associated with the metabolic syndrome (and therefore with errant insulin action), but where the link has not yet been explained in detail: obstructive sleep apnoea and gout.

Obstructive sleep apnoea

Obstructive sleep apnoea is very common in individuals with or without diabetes. There is heavy snoring and typically breathing stops for up to 30 seconds before starting again by itself. In severe cases this cycle is repeated hundreds of times during the night. People with obstructive sleep apnoea are often drowsy during the day and are prone to dropping off to sleep – for example, during meetings, when it is embarrassing, and while driving, when the hazards are obvious. There is no doubt that obstructive sleep apnoea is associated with the metabolic syndrome, and also with severe hypertension and an increased risk of stroke; but in what way insulin and insulin resistance are involved isn't known. Treatment with a face mask during the night, delivering air into the nose and mouth under slight pressure (continuous positive airway pressure, 'CPAP') can be dramatically effective in relieving symptoms and improving quality of life. It was hoped that long-term use might reduce the risk of heart attacks and strokes in sleep apnoea patients who are prone to cardiovascular disease, but a large clinical trial of people with known heart disease did not show any specific benefit after nearly seven years follow-up, possibly because CPAP treatment doesn't consistently reduce blood pressure in these often-hypertensive people.

Gout

Gout is caused by excess uric acid in the circulation that is released near joints, especially the big toe, where it causes inflammation and, reportedly, some of the worst pain imaginable. It can affect other joints, but mostly the hands and feet. In the past it was always thought to be a particular problem of overweight old men who drank too much port, and although an attack can be brought on by drinking too much alcohol, it is very often seen in young people who don't drink. Strangely, cherries can precipitate attacks. Because treatment is so successful, kidney failure, the worst complication of gout, and one which must have resulted in the premature death of thousands of people in the 17th and 18th centuries, is almost never seen, though kidney stones made of uric acid crystals are still very common (they can cause renal colic, another horribly agonising pain). Abnormal insulin is likely to be the culprit, which somehow increases the amount of circulating uric acid. Drug treatment is usually very effective in preventing attacks, but dietary management can help. Although gout itself is very dramatic, in most people with the metabolic syndrome, even though blood uric acid levels are often high, they are not sufficient to cause gout.

Can reducing slightly elevated uric acid levels reduce the risk of heart disease, strokes and kidney impairment? The answer isn't known yet. Formal trials of diet, medication or combinations of these have not been done, and they're not likely to be performed because of the long investigation period, because of the large numbers of participants needed, and because the prototype drug for reducing blood uric acid levels – allopurinol – is now over 60 years old, and so successful (and cheap) that only one additional medication has been launched. However, in people with uric acid kidney stones, careful combinations of medication, diet and specific fluids can be dramatically successful in reducing stone formation.

Other treatments for the metabolic syndrome

A few years ago, there was a flurry of interest in a fatty acid – conjugated linoleic acid – available as a health food supplement for the metabolic syndrome and to help weight loss. One short study showed no benefit, but there's no shortage of speculative 'fat busters', or tablets and electrical treatments for 'boosting metabolism', none of which has a whiff of a proper clinical trial to support its use. Sadly, the same goes for the usual round of highly specific alternative treatments: coconut oil, cayenne pepper, grape seed extract and spinach, among others.

Summary

Formally defined, the metabolic syndrome comprises pre-diabetic blood glucose levels that are not quite normal, but are not yet at levels that define diabetes, together with elevated blood pressure, large waist size and abnormal levels of non-cholesterol lipids (HDL cholesterol and triglycerides). In people with this 'narrow' definition of the metabolic syndrome, some medications and stringent lifestyle interventions can help reduce the rise in blood glucose levels, and weight loss and exercise may have a legacy effect on cardiovascular events that persists for many years after clinical trials have finished. The wider scope of medically relevant conditions encompassed by the metabolic syndrome is increasing; these conditions are not usually associated with pre-diabetes, but all in some way involve abnormal actions of insulin.

Chapter 4

Is Type 2 potentially reversible?

Key points

- Overeating, especially starches, carbohydrates and sugars, results in fat being stored in the liver and pancreas (and other organs too) and causes high blood glucose levels.
- The same process occurs when we overfeed geese, cows and salmon with too much carbohydrate.
- Fat in the liver and pancreas prevents insulin metabolising glucose properly, and blood glucose levels can rise, first to pre-diabetic levels, then to Type 2 levels.
- Fat also gets stored outside and inside the tummy and in muscles. Although these processes don't appear to be central in causing Type 2 in the same way as fatty liver and pancreas, too much tummy fat probably makes diabetes worse because excess fat produces lots of toxic inflammatory chemicals.
- Reducing calorie intake to around 600–800 kcal/day (compared with the usual average of 2000–2500 kcal/day) massively reduces liver fat and probably pancreas fat too. Within a few days of limiting food intake in this way, insulin starts working better, and some of the fundamental abnormalities in Type 2 are reversed. This is the 'Newcastle' diet.
- Evidence is emerging that this is a realistic approach in real life and may help in particular those diagnosed with Type 2 diabetes in the previous six years to go into long-term remission.

A few years ago, a research project from Newcastle University caused great excitement because it showed that severe dieting for six to eight weeks could reverse many of the abnormalities of the liver and pancreas that occur in Type 2, and which were discussed in Chapter 1. The most important of these abnormalities include the tendency of the liver to over-produce glucose, which in turn results from insulin not working efficiently in the liver, and the pancreas failing to produce sufficient insulin. Since then, there has been no shortage of books on how to 'reverse' Type 2 diabetes. There's certainly no magic involved and no effort-free method (we'll discuss the mostly mythical 'superfoods' separately in Chapter 6), but all this research work has given us much more insight into Type 2 diabetes and a new impetus towards non-drug treatment. It has taught us that treating the fundamental abnormalities in Type 2 will themselves reduce blood glucose levels. Simply treating the blood glucose levels – with medication and insulin – does not help the underlying problems (for example, it was widely thought that insulin treatment in particular would help restore the function of the insulin-producing beta cells of the pancreas, but very careful studies have not been able to show this).

Fat in the wrong places in non-human species

Geese: foie gras

The most obvious example of a non-human species that develops fatty liver when overfed is the goose. You will know of – even if you don't approve of – *foie gras* in geese, which has been produced since Roman times. Strangely, or perhaps not so strangely, *foie gras* translates as … fatty liver. If you've seen (or eaten) it, you'll know that it looks off-white or putty-coloured, compared with the dark brown-red colour of normal liver. This is because each liver cell is stuffed with fat.

You'll also know that *foie gras* is produced by force-feeding geese. Again, leaving aside the disquiet that many people have with this process, you might think that producing a fatty liver would require a high *fat* diet. But 2000 years ago the Romans knew that you don't get proper *foie gras* if you feed fat to geese. You need carbohydrate. Today the feed is mostly corn, but the Romans used figs. They didn't understand metabolic pathways, but carbohydrate generates fats called triglycerides – remember in the metabolic syndrome in humans, blood levels of triglycerides tend to be high (see Chapter3). Edible fats eventually find their way into the liver after metabolism, but carbohydrates are the fastest route to fat.

Key point: Fatty liver is caused mostly by over-eating carbohydrates, not fat.

Wagyu *beef: fatty muscle*

If there are a few myths around *foie gras*, then there are whole sagas surrounding *wagyu* beef. These fine animals originate from Japan, but because of high demand for their beef they are now also farmed in Scotland. In this case we are not interested in their livers (though they're very likely to be fatty, just like the geese), but in the muscle. The renowned taste of wagyu beef is due to its high fat content. The fat doesn't surround the meat in a thick layer, but accumulates between sections of the muscle, giving a dramatically 'marbled' appearance. In addition, though we can't see it with the naked eye, there is fat inside the muscle cells themselves.

How is this very expensive meat produced? There's a whole lot of blather about massage and beer, but sadly these measures are needed to calm very stressed animals which spend nearly all their lives housed (there's almost no natural grassland in Japan, so you can't raise free-range animals eating grass and hay). They're fed a diet almost identical to the *foie gras* geese – pure carbohydrate. Adding fats to the diet doesn't change the fat composition of the meat (another indication that what goes in doesn't end up where we might expect).

Farmed salmon

The same processes may be at work in farmed salmon, which has flabby pale pink flesh and – though this is argued – a higher fat content. Wild salmon is firmer, and much more brightly coloured, largely because of the high protein content of the shrimp that are the natural diet of wild salmon.

Humans, animals, and probably fish as well, all have similar metabolic systems that convert extra energy, especially if it's in the form of starchy carbohydrate, into fat which accumulates primarily in the liver and pancreas, and in the tummy and in muscles. The effect of this is to impair the ability of insulin from the pancreas to keep blood glucose levels normal.

The Newcastle research

It's been known for many years that severely restricting food intake lowers blood glucose levels very rapidly in people with Type 2. The experiments of the Newcastle researchers explored two questions:

- First, does restricting food intake in relatively newly diagnosed Type 2s not only reduce blood glucose levels, but also influence the levels of fat in the liver and pancreas – in other words, the two main underlying problems thought to *cause* Type 2?
- Second, if this fat accumulation is the key process in causing Type 2 diabetes, then dietary restriction should improve glucose control in Type 2s no matter how long the individual has had diabetes.

The research that caused so much excitement was published in 2011 in an academic journal (see Reference section on page 213). The title of the research paper, or at least its first five words, made everyone sit up and pay attention: 'Reversal of type 2 diabetes'.

These dramatic words immediately made the headlines, and seven years on, the very appealing word 'reversal' continues to do so. The subtitle ('Normalisation of beta cell function in association with decreased pancreas and liver triacylglycerol') was a touch less catchy, but we can now easily translate it using what we have learned in previous chapters: the pancreas (containing the beta cells that produce insulin) started to work normally, and at the same time fat – triacylglycerol or triglycerides – in both the pancreas and liver decreased. The word 'reversal' is precise and appropriate and conveys the idea of correcting fundamental problems; equally correctly, the word 'cure' doesn't appear anywhere, because that implies a permanent correction. The authors could only make a statement concerning the eight weeks of the study. Of course, this didn't stop the very strong hints in the media about it being a 'cure' for Type 2.

In addition, though, we should recognise this was an experiment – in other words, hardly a real-life study. The 11 participants who had the very low-calorie diet were matched with eight non-diabetic people who were not given any specific advice about dietary restriction. This enabled the researchers to make detailed comparisons between the treated and non-treated group, a standard method used to ensure we know precisely what effects the intervention had. There were multiple blood tests and two magnetic resonance imaging (MRI) scans of the abdomen to measure the amount of fat in the liver and pancreas.

Having said that, the 'treatment' was simple – at least in principle. It was a very low-calorie liquid diet (total 510 kcal/day) supplemented with three portions of non-starchy vegetables (80 kcal/day) to bring the total daily intake to 590 kcal/day. Participants were also encouraged to drink at least two litres of water or other energy-free drinks a day and to keep up their usual levels of exercise. They were intensively supported by nurses, doctors and dieticians throughout the eight-week study. The liquid diet (Optifast, Nestlé) wasn't especially low in carbohydrate (43%), but was high in protein (about one-third), and fat (20%).

Although we are not permitted to know any personal details

of individuals taking part in clinical research studies, their av.. characteristics must always be reported. This helps other clinicians and patients decide whether they could benefit from treatment. In this study, nine of the 11 subjects were men. Their average age was 50, and they had had diabetes for about 2½ years, so they had been diagnosed quite recently. On average they weighed 104 kg (just over 16 stone), and had an average BMI of 34 – that is, very overweight (obesity is BMI of 30 or higher). Blood sugar after fasting overnight was – as expected – 9 mmol/l (recall the non-diabetic value of between 4 and 6).

So … and what happened after taking a very low-calorie diet? After one week:

- Fasting blood glucose fell from 9 to 6 mmol/l – that is, to nearly normal levels – and remained there for the whole eight-week study.
- Glucose output from the liver (remember, usually increased in Type 2 diabetes, and the cause of high glucose levels in the morning) fell to normal.

After eight weeks:

- The overall blood glucose control (measured by HbA_{1c}) fell from 7.4% (58 mmol/mol) to 5.7% (39), again within the non-diabetic range.
- The fat content of the liver fell by two-thirds – back to the level of people who are not overweight and do not have diabetes.
- The fat content of the pancreas fell by 25%.
- The production of insulin from the pancreas increased towards normal.
- Weight fell by 15 kg (nearly 2½ stone), and BMI fell from 34 to 28 ('overweight').

It's hardly surprising that this study caused massive interest: blood glucose normal and weight down by 2½ stones in two months sounds

– and is – remarkable. But we have to remember that 600 kcal food intake every day would feel like near-starvation for most of us, so it's a tribute to the participants and the researchers that this very stringent diet could be maintained for so long. In fact, in the three months after the study had finished, and patients were back to their normal mixed-food diet – though they had received a lot of education about healthy eating – they inevitably regained some weight, but only 3 kg (about ½ stone). Just as important, a repeat MRI showed that fat in the liver and pancreas hadn't changed. In other words, the metabolic machinery had been 'reset' and after three months on a normal low-calorie diet remained in its more efficient state.

Key point: Taking a very low-calorie diet (600 kcal/day) for eight weeks made people with Type 2 very difficult to distinguish metabolically from non-diabetic counterparts.

Do people with a longer duration of Type 2 diabetes have the same outcome?

This was the subject of a second Newcastle study. Can people with longer-duration diabetes do as well with the strict diet as those with more recent-onset diabetes? In summary: most people, even with longer-duration diabetes, show some reversal of their condition with severe dietary restriction, though those with shorter-duration diabetes respond more predictably. The question is of great importance to Type 2s, because it gets to the heart of a widespread view of diabetes – that it is a 'progressive' disorder. I'll discuss this before returning to the Newcastle project.

Type 2 diabetes as a 'progressive' disorder

Twenty years ago, in 1998, a very large and very long clinical trial in newly diagnosed Type 2 people reported its results. This was the famous United Kingdom Prospective Diabetes Study (usually known as UKPDS) (see Reference section, page 214). It was described as 'prospective' because people were followed up from the time of their diagnosis. A major conclusion of the UKPDS was that after the first year of intensive treatment with diet or medication, during which blood glucose levels fell dramatically to not far off normal values (very similar, in fact, to the first Newcastle study), glucose levels progressively rose over the next six to nine years, despite everyone's efforts, to the point at which many participants required insulin treatment. This progression, often known as the UKPDS 'tick', is shown in Figure 4.1.

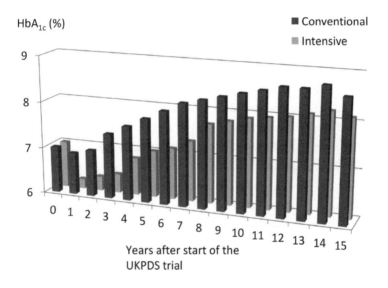

Figure 4.1: A representation of average blood glucose levels in the UKPDS. After an initial sharp fall to nearly normal, they progressively rose over the following 15 years. Conventional treatment was mostly diet-based.

The UKPDS research gave rise to the view, widely accepted, that Type 2 diabetes is a progressive disorder in which blood glucose levels invariably increase with the years. At the same time, the UKPDS investigators found that the basic disorders in Type 2 – the pancreas not producing sufficient insulin and the liver over-producing glucose – seemed to progress at the same rate as blood glucose levels increased. The implication was that it might be more difficult to control blood glucose levels in people with longer-duration diabetes.

This idea also gave rise to two drug-orientated concepts:

- Insulin treatment might be valuable shortly after Type 2 diabetes is diagnosed. The idea is that insulin given by injection helps preserve the function of the pancreas, by 'resting' it (the word is often used). There's *no evidence* for this, but it is widely believed, and promoted, especially in the USA.
- We need to use drugs to get on top of blood glucose levels as soon as they show any sign of increasing (see Chapter 7).

This view – that blood glucose levels generally deteriorate with time and require heavier drug treatment to try and control them – is, however, not currently how Type 2 is viewed – and is definitely not the view of the Newcastle investigators. In general, healthcare professionals and patients are much better at dealing with blood glucose levels than was the case in the 1980s and 1990s, and many studies have shown that keeping blood glucose levels stable is – at least in clinical trials that have gone on for many years – quite feasible, often with minimal medication that by no means invariably progresses to insulin treatment.

Short-duration compared with long-duration diabetes in the Newcastle follow-up study

Let's return to Newcastle. Can their radical eight-week diet treatment with 600 kcal/day 'reverse' Type 2, even in those with many years of diabetes? Some of the patients in their follow-up study had shorter-duration diabetes (average two years, 52 years old); the longer-duration participants had been diagnosed about 13 years previously and had an average age of 62. They had the same degree of overweight as in the first study (average BMI 34, weight nearly 100 kg or 15½ stones).

As in the first study, people with short-duration diabetes all responded well, and fasting glucose levels fell to normal (6.0 mmol/l); in the longer-duration group, starting blood glucose was much higher (13.4 mmol/l) and though the fall was greater, average final glucose level was still higher than in the short-duration group, around 8.0 mmol/l. Around one-half of the longer-duration group had the same excellent response as the short-duration group, but the remaining participants had either a much more sluggish response, or – in about a quarter of them – there was little or no response. Importantly, weight loss was similar in both groups – around 13–15 kg (2–2½ stones), the same as in the original study.

Does blood glucose control remain good even after relaxation of the diet?

This is another question that was tackled in the same follow-up Newcastle study. If a 600 kcal/day liquid diet 'reverses' the liver and pancreas problems associated with diabetes, do people have to continue to take the same liquid diet for diabetes to remain in remission? (Nobody could stick to such a stringent diet in the long term.) After eight diet weeks in the mixed group of short- and longer-duration diabetes, those who had achieved good fasting glucose levels (under 7 mmol/l) were gradually reintroduced to a much more normal diet – a so-called 'isocaloric' diet where one-third of the calories are derived from respectively carbohydrate, fat and protein – though the aim was still to prevent weight regain. On this diet improvements were maintained in all those who responded to the eight-week, very low-calorie diet.

So, the Newcastle approach seems to be generally valuable in newly diagnosed Type 2s, though not so reliably successful in those with longer-duration diabetes. However, even after a long time with diabetes, many patients still had a good response, and this finding contrasts with the idea of Type 2 diabetes as a condition that always progresses.

Does the Newcastle approach work in 'real life'?

Nevertheless, this very radical approach must still be considered experimental and the very low-calorie diets in liquid form are – correctly – only licensed for use under strict medical supervision. Putting this form of diet treatment into widespread practice in real life was the next and rather daunting task enthusiastically taken on by the Newcastle team

The first year results of the DiRECT study (planned to continue for two years in total) were published at the end of 2017 (DiRECT stands for Diabetes REmission Clinical Trial – see Reference section on page 214). In Newcastle and Glasgow over 300 Type 2s were recruited with an average of three years of diabetes. They were similar to the participants in the original trial: their average age was 53, and they were very overweight with an average weight of around 100 kg, giving a body mass index of 35. About one-quarter were on diet alone, while the remainder took medication, but insulin-taking people weren't included.

The target weight loss was 15 kg, as established in the earlier studies, and the aim was to find how many people went into diabetes remission, judged by an HbA_{1c} measurement of 6.5% or less (48 mmol/mol), while taking no diabetes medication. They started with three months of a low-calorie liquid diet containing slightly more energy than in the earlier studies, 800 kcal/day compared with 600. If patients wished, they could continue taking the liquid diet for up to five months. Thereafter, solid food replaced the liquid, and with very careful follow-up, they were encouraged to maintain their lower weight. At this stage they were encouraged to maintain and increase activity levels. As you would expect, the chances of going into diabetes remission for the full year depended on how much weight they managed to lose:

- only 7% went into diabetes remission if weight loss was less than 5 kg
- 34% did so if they managed 5–10 kg weight loss
- 86% did so if they succeeded with 15 kg or more weight loss (see Figure 4.2).

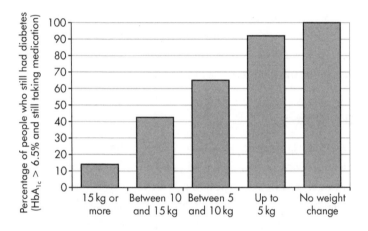

Figure 4.2: Remission of diabetes in the DiRECT study, targeting 15 kg weight loss in Type 2 patients. Only a small number still had diabetes after losing 15 kg or more, while up to 5 kg weight loss was very unlikely to result in remission.

Overall, about one-half completed the year in remission and taking no medication for diabetes. Quality of life improved, while it showed no change in the control group who didn't have the diet. This novel approach is now becoming a practical possibility for large numbers of people, especially those with relatively recent-onset diabetes, in spite of the severity of the diet, so long as their motivation is fully supported.

Key point: Aiming for weight loss of 15 kg will result in about one-half of people with Type 2 going into remission for at least a year, but for the greatest chance of success they must have quite a short duration of known diabetes – less than six years – and not be taking insulin.

Naturally, this isn't the only calorie-restriction approach to managing diabetes; it's just the one that has taken on a life of its own because it has such profound effects on the diabetes process. We'll examine more generally applicable and less stringent diets – which do not result in result in reversal of diabetes, but may still have significant long-term health benefits – in Chapter 5.

Summary

Overeating, especially carbohydrates, is the key to development of fatty liver and probably fatty pancreas. The physiology is not restricted to humans: we overfeed geese, cattle and fish with carbohydrate as well as ourselves, with resulting fat accumulation in liver and within muscle. In human diabetes, very severe dietary restriction to around 600–800 kcal/day for eight weeks rapidly reverses fat accumulation and restores normal fasting glucose. This approach is likely to be more successful in people with shorter-duration diabetes. Many cases of Type 2 diabetes are not irreversible and do not inevitably progress.

Chapter 5

Taking control of calories

Key points

- Weight loss is a major goal of diabetes management.
- Bariatric surgery, resulting in 20–40 kg (3–6 stones) weight loss, often puts Type 2 diabetes into permanent remission, regardless of how long it's been present.
- Losing 15 kg (2 stones) or more (such as with the Newcastle diet – see page 213) can reverse Type 2 diabetes.
- Losing 10 kg (1½ stones) or more over a year reduces the risk of heart attacks (Look AHEAD study – see page 214).
- The benefits of lesser weight loss, such as 5–10 kg (¾ to 1½ stones), aren't so clear: although blood glucose levels probably fall, this may not be sufficient to reduce the risk of long-term complications.
- Changing *what* we eat, especially individual foods, has not been shown to improve long-term outcomes of diabetes – except the Mediterranean diet, which reduces the risk of vascular complications, and possibly also the risk of some cancers.
- Increasing carbohydrate intake and reducing saturated fat – standard dietary advice for Type 2s – is not especially effective in helping weight loss, and has not been shown to improve long-term outcomes.
- Many people find it easier to keep their weight down by reducing carbohydrates and boosting protein intake. Some find intermittent dieting (e.g. the 5:2 diet) quite easy to stick to.
- After losing weight, the risk of regaining it is lower if you eat more protein and low GI carbohydrates, and boost your activity levels (see Chapter 8).

We saw in Chapter 4 that if you cut down your food intake each day from around 2000 kcal to 600-800 kcal then you will lose around 15 kg (2 stone) in eight weeks. In a good proportion of Type 2s, this approach will reduce fasting blood glucose levels to non-diabetic values (4–6 mmol/l), and also restore the liver and pancreas to near-normal. If – if – we could continue this severe reduction in food intake indefinitely, then it's possible that diabetes could remain pretty well permanently reversed. We know this because in 70–80% of people with poor diabetes control who have weight-reducing bariatric/metabolic surgery (for example, a gastric bypass operation), Type 2 stays in remission for a very long time – in some cases nearly 20 years – even in people who were taking insulin treatment. However, weight loss after bariatric surgery is often huge – 30–40 kg (roughly 5–6 stones), two or three times more than is achieved with the Newcastle regimen of consuming 600–800 kcal/day.

We'll address the following questions in this chapter:

- Are there any practical changes we can make to the diet we eat which will reduce the impact of the most serious complications of diabetes – that is, vascular diseases, especially heart attacks, strokes and kidney disorders?
- Is there a portfolio of lifestyle interventions that reduce blood glucose levels and weight in the short and medium term, and the risk of complications in the long term?

We'll start with this last question.

The Look AHEAD clinical trial of weight loss and exercise

The huge Look AHEAD trial (see References, page 214) asked a simple question: Can a really intensive adherence to lifestyle changes, especially weight loss and exercise, reduce the risk of heart attacks and stroke in people with Type 2 diabetes? It's difficult to think of a more ambitious study.

Included were people in their late 50s, with an average of about five years of diagnosed diabetes. About one in eight had had a previous heart attack or stroke. Average weight at the start of the trial was just over 100 kg (15½ stones, BMI nearly 35). You'll recognise these features: they are very similar to those of the Type 2s taking part in the Newcastle studies discussed in the previous chapter (see also page 213). Half of the 5000 participants were given targets of diet, weight loss and exercise, including:

- At least 7% weight loss (that is, 7 kg – just over 1 stone), using a lower-calorie diet of between 1200 and 1800 kcal/ day, depending on body weight. The recommended diet was conventional for the time, focusing on lower fat intake. Participants were encouraged to replace two meals a day with liquid shakes, and one snack with an energy bar.
- Nearly three hours of moderate exercise every week. Activity was mostly extra walking, aiming – as was the vogue at the time – for a minimum of 10,000 steps a day (see Chapter 8).

The other group was given general lifestyle education, but there was no intensive intervention. What happened?

After nearly 10 years of follow-up, there was no reduction in heart attack or stroke rates. Weight loss flattened out at about 8 kg after the first year, but then gradually bounced back – though after eight years there was still about 4 kg loss. (Interestingly, the education given to the non-intensive group seemed to have some effect, because they gradually lost about 2 kg.)

Blood glucose control improved over the first year – though this was a group of people who at the start already had good glucose control (average HbA_{1c} 7.2%, 55 mmol/mol). Blood glucose levels then gradually increased, but after eight years they were no worse than at the start so overall they had held steady. This is quite an achievement if we hold the pessimistic medical view, discussed in Chapter 4, that Type 2 always progresses (it also compares favourably with the outcomes in the UKPDS trial, during which blood glucose control deteriorated to levels much higher than at the start). But if we think along 'Newcastle' lines, was there any evidence for 'remission' of diabetes? In other words, how many Look AHEAD people moved from Type 2 diabetes to pre-diabetes ('partial remission', that is fasting glucose between 5.5 and 6.9 mmol/l) or to normal glucose levels ('full remission', fasting glucose less than 5.5)? Disappointingly, though perhaps not surprisingly, while about 10% had partial or full remission lasting for two years, only about 4% had the same outcome at four years. So, this conventional approach to lifestyle doesn't reverse Type 2.

But all was not negative in Look AHEAD:

- Medication requirements fell – for treatment of blood glucose, cholesterol and blood pressure.
- In those who started with some kidney impairment caused by diabetes, kidney function improved.
- Days in hospital were reduced and symptoms of depression improved.
- People who did especially well with lifestyle intervention, who managed to lose 10 kg in the first year and substantially improve their fitness by 2 METs (see Chapter 8), had fewer cardiovascular events.

Key point: Cardiovascular risk decreases in people who can lose 10 kg and significantly increase their activity over a year. But in most Type 2s, even intensive lifestyle intervention does not reduce glucose levels much, and does not reduce the risk of heart attacks, though important aspects of general health improve.

These are positive messages from the Look AHEAD trial – and there will be further reports following up the participants, even though the trial itself was terminated. But other studies since Look AHEAD have used different approaches, and we can make even more positive suggestions based on their results. This is the point to introduce the Mediterranean diet approach.

The Mediterranean diet

Look AHEAD demonstrated that a moderate lifestyle regimen prevented overall deterioration in blood glucose levels in Type 2 but failed to reduce the long-term concern of cardiovascular risk. Can a different dietary approach reduce vascular events? More specifically, can changes to the *type* of diet, rather than the quantity of food you eat, reduce the risk of serious outcomes?

This really important question gets to the heart (almost literally) of the conundrum of Type 2 diabetes. We are taught that reducing blood glucose levels and keeping them 'low' will reduce the risk of the most serious complications of diabetes (heart attack, stroke and kidney disease). And there is some evidence from a series of major post-UKPDS trials reporting about 10 years ago that very stringent reductions in blood glucose levels (not far off non-diabetic levels, for example 5–6 mmol/l) can, in fact, reduce these events, but only to a limited degree (see page 214). Can we achieve better results by adopting particular diets that concentrate on specific foods to reduce vascular risk without the need specifically to focus on achieving low blood glucose levels?

Key point: Improving blood glucose levels even to near-non-diabetic values has only a limited effect on the important consequences of diabetes, especially heart attacks and strokes, and eye and kidney complications.

The traditional Mediterranean diet

During the 1950s, astute scientists observed that, in spite of a diet containing high levels of fat, people living in southern Europe, for example Italy, Spain and Greece, had much lower risks of vascular diseases than people living in the north. It gradually became apparent that the main reason for this lower risk was the traditional Mediterranean diet. Even more interesting, towards the North Pole it was also found that native arctic Canadians almost never had coronary heart disease although their diet was predominantly fish and seal meat and blubber – that is, very high in 'animal' fat. Medical interest gained momentum in the mid-1990s with the Lyon Heart Study. In this study French people discharged from hospital after a heart attack were allocated either to a Mediterranean diet or to their usual diet. Over the next four years the Mediterranean diet group had a 50–70% lower rate of further heart trouble. At the time, the importance of the central component of the Mediterranean diet – olive oil – wasn't appreciated, nor the critical importance of omega 3 fatty acids in fish (and the mammals whose diet was fish), but the Mediterranean diet train had already started its journey. In the early 2000s a huge study in Greece found that people who stuck closely to the traditional Mediterranean diet had the lowest risk of heart attack and strokes, though any degree of adherence was associated with a lower risk than those who didn't stick to it at all. This result came as no great surprise to cardiologists, but a more unexpected finding was that cancer risk was also reduced by a Mediterranean diet – and the more components of the diet people kept to, the lower the risk.

Key point: The traditional Mediterranean diet is strongly associated with a lower risk of heart attack, stroke and some forms of cancer.

The PREDIMED study

Fast forward 15 years to 2013, when the results of a modern study of the Mediterranean diet were published. Nearly half of the people in the Spanish PREDIMED study (see References, page 217) had Type 2. Participants were allocated for five years to a strict Mediterranean diet, or the same Mediterranean diet supplemented with either 1 litre a week of extra-virgin olive oil, or 30 g mixed nuts daily. It's important to remember that the trial wasn't concerned with achieving weight loss. Participants could eat what they wanted, so long as they stuck to the Mediterranean diet and their extra supplement, olive oil or nuts. In the people with Type 2, there was no special attempt to reduce blood glucose, blood pressure or cholesterol levels: these matters were left to the usual medical teams of the participants.

The recommended diet is shown in Table 5.1. It's worth looking at it in detail; it reminds us that the traditional Mediterranean diet is mostly a home-cooked diet. It goes without saying that 'traditional Mediterranean' does not include an occasional plate of spaghetti with commercial bottled and high-sugar 'Bolognese', sauce, supersized stuffed-crust take-away pizza, or double-cream gelato with added sprinkles and fluorescent syrups. How many of the recommendations do you stick to, and how many could you incorporate into your everyday life? (I didn't even know of the existence of sofrito until recently, yet this marvellous mixture of vegetables and olive oil is a good example of a great Mediterranean ingredient you'd barely notice when served in a soup or pasta sauce.)

Table 5.1: Mediterranean diet recommended in the PREDIMED study

Recommended	Target consumption
Extra-virgin olive oil	4 or more tablespoonsful a day (with a further 4–8 in total – in the group taking additional olive oil)
Nuts and peanuts	3 or more servings a week (30 g or 1 ounce daily in the group assigned to additional nuts: ½ ounce walnuts, ¼ ounce each of almonds and hazelnuts)
Fresh fruits	3 or more servings a day
Vegetables	3 or more servings a day
Fish (especially fatty/oily), seafood	3 or more servings a week
Legumes (beans)	3 or more servings a week
Sofrito	2 or more servings a week (sofrito is a traditional Italian base for pasta sauces and soups, consisting of finely chopped carrots, celery and onions cooked very slowly in olive oil)
White meat	In place of red meat
Wine	7 or more glasses a week (optional, only for people who normally drank alcohol)
Discouraged	**Target limits**
Soft drinks	Fewer than 1 drink a day
Commercial bakery foods, sweets and pastries	Fewer than 3 servings a week
Spread fats	Fewer than 1 serving a day
Red and processed meats	Fewer than 1 serving a day

What were the results of the PREDIMED study?

- People with diabetes and those without had the same outcomes.
- There was a 30% reduction in cardiovascular events in both the nut and extra-virgin olive oil groups.

- People in the olive oil group had a lower overall death rate.
- Better brain function.
- Weight and waist circumference fell slightly in the olive oil group but not the nut-supplemented group.
- Mediterranean diet with extra olive oil (but not nuts) may protect against diabetic eye disease (retinopathy, see Chapter 11).

Key point: Incorporate extra-virgin olive oil into your diet wherever you can.

PREDIMED is a very important study for people with Type 2 diabetes. There's no mention of drugs, insulin treatment, 'aggressive' attempts to reduce blood glucose, blood pressure or even keeping weight down. The reductions in risk of vascular disease and death were due solely to adherence to a strict Mediterranean diet with a large addition of extra-virgin olive oil. Some benefits were seen with nuts, but the best outcomes were with the olive oil. It can't be any old form of olive oil. It must be extra-virgin. But remember, this is a 'portfolio' solution where multiple dietary components, combined with extra-virgin olive oil, gave astonishing results.

It's not clear whether the startling benefits of extra-virgin olive oil relate to its very high monounsaturated fatty acid levels, or – as is suspected, but not known for certain – the fruit-derived chemicals, the polyphenols, that give extra-virgin olive oil its wonderful bright green colour, and its pungent and very peppery flavour.

For northern Europeans, the problem is that olive oil isn't an integral part of our diet culture; it's seen more as a luxury addition. But there are many ways we can integrate it more fully into our diet. In Italy, when food arrives the first thing the Italians do – including the youngsters who order pizza – is reach for the bottle of olive oil that's always sitting on the restaurant table. They'll pour a huge amount, perhaps 20 ml (2 tablespoonsful) on their food, almost regardless of what they ordered. While we may not be able to do that every day in the UK, the box below includes some suggestions for supplementing your olive oil intake.

Simple ways to incorporate more extra-virgin olive oil into our diet

- Try grilling vegetables – and then add more extra-virgin olive oil before serving.
- If frying vegetables, use half olive oil and half your usual cooking oil.
- Drizzle olive oil onto bread (of any kind) you eat with soups and salads.
- Instead of butter, drizzle olive oil onto breakfast toast to eat with ham, fish, eggs or salads. This is much more 'natural' and tastes better than olive oil-based spreads, which contain a feeble amount of actual olive oil (only about 15–20%), together with other oils. Although the ingredient lists don't state what quality olive oil is used in spreads, it won't be extra-virgin, so even if you could eat huge amounts, it probably wouldn't deliver the PREDIMED health benefits.
- Always use olive oil (and good quality vinegar, especially real balsamic) for salad dressings.
- Snack on green olives, even though individually they don't contain much oil. Black olives, though tasty, contain little oil. Perhaps 20–40 small green olives will provide about 1 tablespoonful of oil. So, snacking on green olives probably won't boost your oil intake that much, but they're likely to be better than many other snack options.
- Don't forget an ounce of nuts daily. Although the combined effects of extra olive oil and nuts were not studied in PREDIMED, we know the benefit of nuts alone was substantial.

In summary, we can describe dietary approaches to Type 2 diabetes in a clear way:

- The Newcastle approach reverses Type 2 diabetes. Presumably if people could stick to it for years there would be a reduction in cardiovascular disease – though we don't know that for certain.
- The strict Mediterranean diet with additional extra-virgin olive oil reduces cardiovascular disease (and possibly cancer) without any need to specifically focus on blood glucose levels (we don't even know what happened to weight, blood glucose or blood pressure in the PREDIMED participants with Type 2).
- The standard weight loss diet with high carbohydrates and low saturated fat, together with moderate exercise, prevents blood glucose levels getting worse, but doesn't reduce cardiovascular outcomes (Look AHEAD).

Lower carbohydrate, higher protein diets

Lower carbohydrate diets are very popular and have been for nearly 20 years. They seem to be as effective for losing weight as any other diet, but they are easier to sustain. The vogue began in the early 2000s with the extremely low-carbohydrate Atkins diet. Atkins's original idea – incorrect, as it turned out – was that low carbs would cause weight loss because the body required more of its own energy to metabolise fat than carbohydrate. Atkins's arbitrary plan, based on no science at all, was that in the initial phase of the diet people should eat no more than about 20 g carbohydrate a day, gradually increasing to 50 g daily over about six months (compared with about 200 g in a normal diet). These were punitively low carbohydrate amounts (20 g is two very small slices of bread), and almost impossible to sustain. Variants of Atkins soon joined the low-carb bandwagon, including the Dukan diet, the Zone diet, the South Beach diet, and latterly

Paleo diet. They've all had their vogue and, like all diets, if they'd worked the magic they promised we wouldn't need the next fad.

There were no proper clinical trials of Atkins-like diets (certainly none in Type 2 people), and there was concern about possible adverse effects of eating such minuscule quantities of carbohydrate, together with very high amounts of protein and, in the case of meat, associated fat intake. But Atkins got people thinking about the wisdom of the standard dietary advice we had been giving everyone, including Type 2s, for decades – and for which there was almost no evidence either. You'll be aware of the advice because if you've seen a dietician in the past you're likely to have been given it: lots of carbohydrates and as little fat as possible. The reasons behind it were that high carbohydrate intake wasn't seen to be harmful, but that 'fat' caused arterial thickening and thereby increased the risks of heart attacks and strokes. I'll discuss the fat controversy below, but let's start with the 'high carbohydrates are good' part.

Some doctors and many people with diabetes thought advising a high carbohydrate intake was a bit strange when – as we know – carbohydrates are broken down very quickly and can cause high glucose peaks shortly after eating them. People with Type 1 diabetes were advised to take up to 60% of their diet as carbohydrates, though in real life they couldn't even manage 50%. They realised that taking a lot of carbohydrate meant taking a lot of insulin, and they quickly understood that even the most 'modern' fast-acting insulin preparations weren't efficient enough to reduce blood glucose levels after a high-carbohydrate meal. The same thought occurred to people with Type 2 taking insulin: the more carbohydrate they ate, the more insulin they needed, leading to increased risks of hypoglycaemia and weight gain. We've also seen in Chapter 4 that carbohydrates fuel fatty liver and probably fatty pancreas as well, both of which are fundamental problems in Type 2. So could a lower-carbohydrate diet have the same long-term benefits as PREDIMED, with no change in calorie intake?

The DiRECT Study: low-carbohydrate diet without specific calorie restriction

DiRECT (2008 – see Refences, page 217) was another good study in people not specifically chosen to have diabetes, this time lasting two years. It tested a low-carbohydrate diet that didn't aim at weight loss. It was done around the time of peak enthusiasm for Atkins, so in the early part of the trial ultra-low carbohydrates were recommended (20 g a day), increasing to 120 g a day, which is low, but not too punitive for most people (I'll give a couple of examples of 120 g below). Average weight loss was quite impressive at nearly 5 kg (11 lb), though remember this is much less than the Newcastle weight loss, and unlikely to 'reverse' Type 2.

The weight loss resulted from participants eating around 400 fewer calories a day. So simply advising people to reduce their carbohydrate intake causes weight loss. Only a small number of people in this trial had Type 2. Blood glucose levels didn't fall (hinting that even 5 kg weight loss may not have a meaningful effect on blood glucose). We don't have data on long-term blood glucose control, measured with HbA_{1c}. This degree of weight loss, although impressive, doesn't seem to have any specific effects on glucose levels, and of course the trial wasn't long enough to examine any effects on diabetes complications. From the Look AHEAD results it's unlikely to be of long-term benefit.

Nevertheless, the study was particularly interesting because the unlimited low-carbohydrate diet was compared with two calorie-restricted diets. One was the Mediterranean diet, which gave about the same weight loss – 5 kg – as the low-carbohydrate diet. However, the standard weight-loss diet (lower calories and low fat) was less successful (3 kg loss), another indication that the traditional recommendations aren't maximally beneficial. You might expect the cholesterol and triglyceride levels to improve more with the low-fat diet, but they didn't: all results were better with the Mediterranean and low-carbohydrate diets. These results should come as no surprise to you with your new knowledge of metabolism: triglycerides are derived mostly from carbohydrates and not fat, and whatever cholesterol there is in food doesn't translate into higher cholesterol in the blood (see Chapter 10).

Why does a lower-carbohydrate diet help weight loss, even though there's no specific restriction on total calorie intake? There are several reasons, not yet supported by evidence from clinical trials, but nonetheless plausible:

- First, lower carbohydrate intake genuinely seems to keep ravenous hunger under control. Many people report that although they *are* hungry when they restrict carbohydrates, they can still manage their hunger without resorting to drastic emergency tactics, such as fridge-raiding or frequent snacking.

- Second, the 'rules' for restricting carbohydrate are quite simple: for most people remembering to cut down bread, potatoes, rice, pasta, cakes and biscuits is straightforward. Compare the kerfuffle of consulting food packaging labels for nutritional details, particularly when you're in a rush and grabbing something pre-packed for lunch. If it's covered in bread, it's likely to be high-carbohydrate (we'll mention this again in Chapter 6, but a standard slice of bread these days weighs in at around 50 g. Two slices, in a standard pre-packed sandwich is therefore already 100 g, and that's without the breakfast cereal, pasta for dinner ... you get the point).

However, it's important to recognise that there is nothing magical about carbohydrate; in another important study (DIOGENES – see References, page 217) people got the same weight loss by reducing fat or protein. But I think the simple diet rule and lack of gnawing hunger together make the low-carbohydrate diet different.

**Example of moderate carbohydrate intake (120 g)
a lower-carbohydrate diet** (Data from Chris Cheyette ar.
Yello Balolia, *Carbs and Cals: Carb and Calorie Counter* 2016;
Chello Publising.)

Breakfast or lunch: 2 slices of medium-sliced white or brown bread (note: same calories and no difference in fibre content)	26 g
Lunch or dinner: medium portion of spaghetti or rice	54 g
Snack: 2 digestive biscuits	20 g
1 pint of beer or lager (4% alcohol by volume, ABV)	17 g
Total	120 g

OR you can blow the whole lot (and a bit more) on a
McDonald's meal:

Hamburger	30 g
Regular milkshake	68 g
Regular fries	42 g
Total	140 g (total calories 970)

Key point: Eating less carbohydrates helps weight loss,
reduces peak blood glucose levels after meals and is
acceptable to many people because it doesn't cause
ravenous hunger. It also improves the blood lipid profile.

Higher protein diets

Most people embarking on lower-carbohydrate diets boost their
protein intake. There aren't many scientific studies of higher-
protein diets, but the DIOGENES study in 2010 found that after

weight loss (eight weeks of an 800 kcal liquid diet), a combination of increased protein and lower glycaemic index (GI) food – see below – prevented weight gain more effectively than the other diets studied. Protein content was doubled up to about 25% of total energy with a combination of lean meat, low-fat dairy products and vegetable protein (beans, peas, lentils).

> **Key point:** To reduce the risk of weight gain after losing weight, double your protein consumption, eat more low-GI carbs, especially wholegrains, lower your carbohydrate intake and make that determined effort to increase activity levels.

Low glycaemic index (GI) foods

We've seen that even if you don't deliberately reduce your food intake, aiming for a lower-carbohydrate diet should help you lose weight. But can eating different *kinds* of carbohydrate also have an effect? This introduces the concept of the glycaemic index (GI) which has been around a long time, and is well established in the diet world. The GI number gives a rough idea of how high blood glucose will rise after eating a particular carbohydrate compared with glucose or white bread – both of which are very rapidly absorbed. Low GI carbohydrates – which give a smaller rise in blood glucose – are widely promoted as 'good' because they are thought to be 'slow release'. Measuring GI is complicated, and the numbers can be hard to interpret, since we don't usually eat one pure carbohydrate alone, and other food types, especially protein, can effectively lower GI. A big deal is often made of small differences. For example, banana has a higher GI than apple – but can avoiding bananas make any meaningful difference to glucose levels or weight? Not according to the one good trial I could find (see References, page 218). In Type 2s studied for a year there were no meaningful differences in either weight or blood glucose control between groups taking a high-GI or a low-GI diet, though glucose control at the start was very good (average HbA$_{1c}$ 6.2%). With the low-GI diet you would expect the peak level of glucose after meals to be lower, but this wasn't seen.

Admittedly, this is only one trial (others are planned), but I can't see much value in debating, for example, whether we should be eating rye crispbread (high GI) or rye pumpernickel (low GI), considering most people (in the UK, at least) don't eat very much of either. Similarly, I don't believe that taking a bowl of porridge for breakfast (usually quoted as the ultimate low-GI 'slow-release' food) can itself improve glucose control (see Figure 5.1). I think GI has focused us on the not very helpful idea that individual food products are 'good' or 'bad'. Individual foods are often minor components in our complex diets. Focusing on globally reducing carbohydrate intake, and increasing Mediterranean-ism is simpler and more effective.

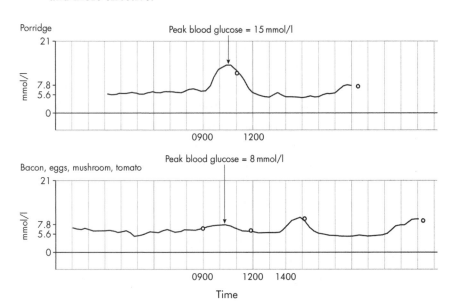

Figure 5.1: Blood glucose responses to breakfasts: porridge and a zero-carb breakfast, both at 0900.

Figure 5.1 is from a person with Type 2, well-controlled on tablets, and shows his blood glucose responses using a personal continuous glucose monitoring system (FreeStyle Libre, Abbott). The upper tracing shows what happened when he ate porridge: blood glucose level rose from 7 mmol/l fasting to peak at 16, and didn't return to baseline levels for about four hours. This doesn't look much like 'slow-release' to me, though you may disagree. However, we can all agree on the interpretation of the lower tracing, which shows a flat-line response to a zero-carb breakfast (bacon, eggs, mushroom, tomato). Blood glucose levels didn't rise at all (the blip later on in the day was caused by a carb-containing lunch). I am grateful to the patient (a 68-year-old man with two years of diabetes) for allowing me to use these informative recordings.

Whole grains versus GI

Whole grains are a key part of the Mediterranean diet, so we'd expect good outcomes in people eating foods containing them. This was confirmed in a huge group of nurses and doctors studied between 1984 and 2010, where death rates from heart disease were 10% lower in those taking a diet containing a lot of whole grains. Note that low GI is quite different from whole grains. Spotting the difference is quite easy: low GI is usually advertised in large letters on a food package, while whole grains can only be detected by the eye (or sometimes the teeth). The British Dietetic Association recommends the following wholegrain foods that are also considered low GI. You'll immediately spot it's quite a short list:

- rolled oats
- wholegrain muesli (not many of these are available unless you make your own)
- bread and crackers (whole grain with multi-grain); seeded, mixed-grain, soya, linseed, rye (pumpernickel)
- wholewheat pasta, whole barley, bulgur (cracked) wheat, quinoa, barley (but not pearl).

Chapter 5

Intermittent fasting (for example the 5:2 diet)

Intermittent fasting regimes are popular at the moment. Restricting food intake one or more days a week is intuitively sound, and chimes with the idea of 'feast and famine' in our ancestry. There are countless variants of intermittent fasting. The most popular is the 5:2 diet where two days a week you eat normal but small meals (total daily calorie intake 500–600 kcal, occasionally 800) – and not to overeat when you return to your normal diet on the remaining five days. It amounts to an average daily calorie deficit of around 400 kcal, which is similar to the amount we saw in the low-carbohydrate diet group of the DiRECT study discussed earlier. Alternate day 'fasting', and daily eating only between certain hours, for example between 10.00 am and 6.00 pm, are also promoted.

There are no major trials of intermittent fasting, but it seems to have no advantages over restricting calories every day, and it has the same drop-out rate (about one in three). There is no evidence that there are benefits beyond the simple reduction in calories: fasting on certain days has no magical significance. As with all diets, it suits some people very well, and they can maintain it over a long period (I'd find myself continually postponing fasting days). There are very intriguing studies in mice and rats where fasting of this kind has been shown to increase life expectancy, but doing the human studies may take some time.

Countless other 'rules' and must-dos and don'ts that are related to times of eating have no good evidence to support them. One is the widespread belief that breakfast is the most important meal of the day (a view promoted 100 years ago by a certain Dr Kellogg). In kids, eating breakfast may be important, as it reduces snacking later in the day. Late dinners are increasingly part of the lives of working adults, but they are probably not harmful, so long as you are not over-compensating for the very long time since lunch.

Commercial weight management programmes

These have always been popular, perhaps even more so now with their online profiles. In addition, they genuinely seem to work, with average weight losses around 5–7 kg (11–15 lb) over six to 12 months (this was in a comparison between Weight Watchers, Rosemary Conley, Atkins and Slimfast diets). However, as always, these averages don't tell the full story. Everyone responds differently. Some people – those on the internet, social media and adverts – do very well, with up to 20 kg weight loss, but we hear less about those who lose almost nothing, or even gain a small amount, and this variation is the same with all the diets. Despite the different methods they use (meal replacements, meal delivery, very low-calorie diets) they all have the same aims – helping people to moderately reduce their food intake and to maintain the reduction. They achieve weight loss more effectively than weight management programmes in the NHS, probably because contact is more frequent, and the resulting motivation higher.

What effect do these diets have on blood glucose control in diabetes?

Losing 10 kg (22 lb, 1½ stone) or more in Look AHEAD had valuable cardiovascular benefits, but remarkably little is known about the impact of more modest degrees of weight loss, say 5–7 kg. Cholesterol and other lipid levels, and blood pressure, show only very small reductions with this degree of weight loss, and may not be noticeable in individuals, and there's amazingly little known about the effect on glucose values.

Scrutinising a few old studies, it looks as if 5 kg weight loss (11 lb) reduces fasting glucose levels by about 1.5 mmol/l (e.g. from 9.0 to 7.5 mmol/l, or 7.5 to 6.0) and HbA_{1c} by about 1.0%. And this takes us to a controversy that shows no sign of going away.

What is the value of small reductions in blood glucose levels?

If you reduce blood glucose levels by 1.5 mmol/l, or reduce HbA_{1c} by 1% through losing 5 kg, is that likely to be of value? As always, the answer depends on whether we're talking about short-term or longer-term benefits. Although the effort involved in losing 5 kg weight results in only modest improvements in blood glucose control, we shouldn't ignore them: one blood glucose-lowering drug may have around the same effect. So, in the short term, you are likely to be able to ditch one of your diabetes drugs, an important consideration (see Chapter 7). But looking to the longer term, the blood glucose effect of around 5 kg weight loss (and therefore the equivalent of a single diabetes medication) is not so impressive. Based on the results of most of the major clinical trials (most of which used medication to reduce glucose levels), changes of this order only slightly reduce the risk of eye and kidney complications; after a long period, perhaps 10 years or more, a few of them found that major vascular events (heart attacks and strokes) were reduced too.

However, we can achieve a greater impact on long-term cardiovascular complications more easily and effectively by reducing blood pressure by about 10 mm or by reducing LDL cholesterol by 1 mmol/l (see Chapter 10). Actually, of course, we should be doing all three, because a simple medication and lifestyle 'portfolio' approach reduces nearly all complications of Type 2, *and* reduces the risk of premature death from cardiovascular disease, *and* prolongs life by an average of seven years (this was the Steno-2 study – see References, page 216) – in people with the earliest indication of diabetic kidney disease). We now have evidence that the 'lifestyle portfolio' of the Mediterranean diet also reduces the risk of important vascular complications – without necessarily improving blood glucose, blood pressure or cholesterol control (we're not sure about that, because as I've already mentioned we don't have this information in Type 2s participating in PREDIMED). However, we can be certain that the two combined portfolios will benefit Type 2s in the long term.

> **Key point:** We can probably achieve the best long-term outcomes in Type 2 diabetes by combining a modest medication portfolio (see Chapter 7) with substantial weight loss and the Mediterranean diet.

The end of the low saturated fat diet?

However, let me now spend a little time on the question of dietary fat, especially saturated fat, because the high-carbohydrate, low saturated fat diet that's been central to dietary advice for people with and without diabetes is – or should be – having a crisis of confidence: science is gently nibbling away at it.

Saturated fat is bad, or that's what we've been told for many years, to the point where in the UK many people actively avoid butter, full-cream milk and cheese. As we've seen, butter has been replaced with olive oil spreads, even though their actual olive oil content is low, and isn't extra-virgin oil, where the health benefits lie. Full-cream milk, even though it contains less than 5% saturated fat (5% is 'low-fat') is often regarded as a lethal additive to tea. But the evidence linking saturated fat intake with heart disease is remarkably weak, and is based on a few small studies that are more than 50 years old. More recently, there have been some good studies that have confirmed again this very weak link, and in 2015 formal dietary advice in the USA did not set limits on the amount of fat in the diet. Although part of the rationale was the weak link between saturated fat intake and heart disease, there were also concerns that a general plea to 'reduce fat' would also prevent people eating mono- and polyunsaturated fats which are universally considered to be protective against heart disease. Predictably, there was a furore when the report was issued.

A massive study – named PURE (PURE standing for Prospective Urban Rural Epidemiology) – was published in 2017 (see References, page 218). It carefully assessed the diet of 130,000 50-year-olds in 18 widely differing countries, and followed them up for about seven years, focusing on heart attacks and strokes. It found that high carbohydrate intakes were associated with an *increased* overall death rate, though not with heart attack or stroke rates. Even more striking were the findings on fat intake. There'll be no surprise that those who ate the most monounsaturated and polyunsaturated fats had the lowest overall mortality: they are the most 'Mediterranean-diet' people. But those who ate more saturated fat had a *lower* stroke rate. The authors were clear: there's no evidence that we should, as conventionally taught, reduce saturated fat intake to less than 10% of total intake. On the contrary, *increasing* total fat intake to around 35% of our total intake (emphasising mono- and polyunsaturated fats), and *lowering* carbohydrate intake, might have long-term health benefits.

Higher carbs risk shortening your life? And saturated fats protecting you against stroke? It's counterintuitive and not at all what we were brought up to believe. Although a single study, however large, shouldn't change anything immediately, there's no longer any need to consider carbohydrates as the basis of our diet and we shouldn't be avoiding fats of any kind. (Remember, though, that large amounts of red meat, especially processed meat, for many of us a major source of saturated fat, probably carry different long-term health problems, especially higher risks of some cancers.)

Key point: While always emphasising monounsaturated and polyunsaturated fats, there is probably no longer any need to limit fat intake. High carbohydrate intake is probably more hazardous than high fat.

Summary

Low-carbohydrate diets are easier to stick to than standard higher-carbohydrate low-saturated-fat diets. They probably have meaningful effects on overall blood glucose levels. A more traditional Mediterranean diet with additional extra-virgin olive oil *does* have benefits – reduced vascular events, and possibly a lower risk of some cancers. Limiting our total fat intake is probably unwise, and saturated fat is only weakly linked to heart disease. Preventing weight regain after weight loss is very difficult, but a combination of higher-protein intake, low-GI carbohydrates and wholegrains and increased activity levels offer the best hope. Modest weight loss can help us reduce our medication burden by reducing blood glucose levels a little, though this does not translate to improved long-term vascular outcomes, unless you can lose 10 kg or more.

Chapter 6

'Superfoods' and nutraceuticals

Key points

- Superfoods claim to reduce blood glucose levels, reduce weight, reduce the risk of heart attacks and even prolong life.
- Nutraceuticals and superfoods are broadly the same, but nutraceutical is the word usually used by professionals, and they've often been tested in the laboratory – usually in the test-tube or in animals. Almost none have been tested adequately in humans.
- Whichever term is used, there's very little evidence that any of them are medically effective.
- But if any nutraceuticals or superfoods are low carbohydrate and fit in with the Mediterranean diet (for example, bitter melon, okra) then eat them for that reason (and because they taste good).
- Vinegar taken with meals may reduce peak blood glucose levels.
- Vitamins, minerals and trace elements don't help, probably because very few of us are really deficient in them, and the body is designed to retain only a minimum amount. Like everything in excess, they can be toxic.
- A mega-trial exploring the vascular effects of cocoa extract is up and running.

The 'superfood' idea is new, and has no strict definition (out of millions of scientific articles, I could find only 17 that had 'superfood' in the title). The medical term – 'nutraceutical' – is much more widely used (70,000 references). Both are used to describe foods or substances extracted from food that may have medically beneficial effects. Although superfoods and nutraceuticals are similar, superfoods have almost never been subjected to scientific studies and are mostly food fashions heavily promoted as having some medical-like benefits. On the other hand, nutraceuticals have often been studied in the laboratory, sometimes very extensively. Most studies are in test-tubes, and some of them in animals, but even though some of the chemicals are biologically impressive and hold out hope that they will be of value in conditions like Type 2 diabetes, almost none have been clinically tested in humans, mostly because it is very difficult to patent these natural substances.

Claims for the health benefits of superfoods are widely promoted, and include weight loss, lowering cholesterol levels and reducing blood glucose levels in Type 2. Additional claims for some include reduced risk of heart disease and Alzheimer's, and even anti-ageing and reducing the risk of cancer. Some are macronutrients – that is, food products that form a large part of our diet – for example, protein or carbohydrate. Examples here would be 'white meat' (contrasted with 'red meat') or 'fruit'. However, usually they are individual food items, mostly specific vegetables or fruits (often berries). Sometimes they are grouped together as menu items, such as 'superfood salad'. Then there is a very interesting group of individual plants, spices and herbs that contain fascinating substances with blood-glucose-lowering effects, though frustratingly there are no clinical trials sufficiently large to be convincing. The exceptions here are guanidine and galegine, blood glucose-lowering chemicals from which metformin was developed, and which were originally isolated from a flowering plant, Goat's rue. Finally, there is a huge group of minerals, trace elements and vitamins that are widely believed to have specific anti-diabetic properties.

I'd like to have space to discuss all the superfoods/nutraceuticals, but this topic alone would require a huge book, so I'll take a few examples that happened to be in vogue while I was writing this chapter. I'll use the background from earlier chapters to help us assess pros and cons, and hopefully equip you to assess the next generation of claims when they arrive, as they most surely will.

> **Key point:** Nutraceuticals are foods, food products or substances contained in food that have biological effects when tested in the laboratory. Superfoods are popular versions of nutraceuticals. Promoted as having medical benefits, they have rarely been studied scientifically.

Using our new knowledge of diabetes to assess 'superfoods'

Let's step back from all the arguments about which superfood is more super than the last, and return to the concepts we discussed in previous chapters. The body tries to digest and then use everything we eat and does so very efficiently, but recall that nearly all the food that can be absorbed into the bloodstream is converted sooner or later to glucose, which is stored or used under the watchful eye of brilliant insulin produced by the pancreas.

The avocado

Let's take the avocado, a 'superfood' from 2016 onwards – at the time of writing a 'megafood' that's become so popular in the West that it was blamed for adverse environmental and economic effects in Mexico where it is a major fruit crop. (This is often the case with popular superfoods, and is another reason why we should always carefully consider the pros and cons of these foods.) Medically, though, could avocado, eaten in sufficient quantities, provide enough healthy monounsaturated fats to give the same benefits as extra-virgin olive oil in the PREDIMED study described in Chapter 5? One myth we can dispatch immediately is that avocados are full of 'cholesterol': only animals synthesise cholesterol, so it forms no part of any plant. Avocados are not high-cholesterol; they are zero-cholesterol. A whole avocado (without its stone) weighs about 150 grams. Here's a table of the components of two whole avocados – a big portion, so it would likely be in a large salad, or perhaps guacamole, but I wouldn't want to be accused of being mean.

Table 6.1 Components of avocado

Nutrient	Proportion	Actual amount contained in two avocados
Water	73%	220 ml (two thirds of a standard drink can)
Fat	15%	45 g
Carbohydrate	5%	15 g
Protein	2%	6 g

- Although avocado is a fruit, it's green and like leafy vegetables it contains folic acid.
- Water – we can all agree – doesn't have any effect on glucose or any aspect of food metabolism. A glass of tap water would be cheaper and involve fewer air miles.
- Carbohydrates, we can see, are very low, so this would, like all vegetables, be a good part of a low-carbohydrate diet. (Avocados don't grow in Mediterranean countries, so, although they would go well with the Mediterranean diet, they aren't 'officially' part of it.)
- Protein – there are tiny amounts which we can ignore.
- What about the fat? Yes, it's mostly monounsaturated and polyunsaturated fat, so it possibly behaves a little like good old olive oil. There are no trials of the benefits of avocado on glucose levels or heart attack rates – and there will never be; but let's make the big assumption, for which there is no evidence, that the healthy fats in avocados have the same

beneficial cardiac effects as the healthy fats in extra-virgin olive oil. In PREDIMED you needed at least a litre every week of extra-virgin olive oil. Simple arithmetic, then: 1 litre of olive oil weighs about 1000 g (1 kg). How many avocados do you need to eat to consume a litre of avocado oil? The answer – 45. Unless you eat 45 or more avocados a week you wouldn't get the health benefits of olive oil supplementation, even if the oils in avocado were equally beneficial (which is most unlikely).

Conclusion: Avocados are not 'superfoods' in the quantities usually eaten, and by themselves can have no health benefits, though they are a good (but small) component of a healthy diet.

> **Key point:** Avocados contain unsaturated fatty acids similar to those in olive oil, but in much smaller amounts. They're nice to eat, but have no special health benefits.

It's strange that while nice-tasting and fashionable fruits such as avocados are often cited as 'superfoods', they don't seem to be of much value, and other more ordinary products, for which there is more plausible evidence, never make it into the headlines. Examples here are lady's fingers (okra) and bitter melon, both cheap and tasty vegetables, and which potentially have a role in lowering blood glucose levels.

Okra

Okra ('ladies' fingers') is widely used as a diabetes treatment in countries where it is eaten as a vegetable. There are good reasons why it may have some effect on blood glucose levels. First, it is high in soluble fibre, which is why it's gooey when cooked. Soluble fibre reduces blood glucose, and a pure soluble fibre, guar gum, was in vogue in the 1980s and 1990s as a prescription drug in Type 2, though you needed to take a large amount each day (around 15 g), and even a good portion of okra (100 g, 3½ ounces) contains much less, perhaps 6 g. However, okra also contains a specific chemical that reduces the amount of glucose absorbed from the gut (very much like a drug called acarbose, a natural product derived from a bacterium, which was also popular 15–20 years ago). Okra may also lower cholesterol and blood pressure (see the section on the DASH diet in Chapter 7), but because there are no clinical trials, we can only recommend it as a very good vegetable in the general diet. Remember also that, like medication, if okra did have good effects on blood glucose, you'd need to eat it every day. Even the keenest okra consumer might have a bit of a problem achieving this. The daily routine obviously applies to all nutraceuticals.

Bitter melon ('karela' in India)

The bitter melon (karela), widely eaten in Indian and south-east Asian cuisines, is also used in traditional medicine as an anti-diabetic agent. In some ways it is similar to okra: it has even higher levels of soluble fibre, and also contains active blood glucose-lowering chemicals which have been isolated and studied in the laboratory. One of these substances works at the point on the cell surface where insulin molecules bind – the insulin receptor. It increases the efficiency of the receptor, and therefore increases uptake of glucose from the circulation and reduces blood glucose levels. It also contains a fascinating substance that inhibits certain natural steroids, and which was seriously investigated by drug companies a few years ago as potentially a very effective blood glucose-lowering drug.

But – critical question – is bitter melon meaningfully effective in reducing blood glucose levels, and how much of this genuinely bitter food do you need to consume? As usual, these are the really difficult questions and unfortunately there are no well-conducted clinical trials. Until these trials are done – and holding our breath until they are may not be a wise strategy here – it should, like okra, be considered a valuable vegetable to include in the diet. Again, the portfolio approach is probably the best: increase the amounts you eat of these entirely safe vegetables, thereby gaining the benefits of the high-vegetable and high-fibre diet, while they possibly have some effect in reducing blood glucose levels. But low glucose level – hypoglycaemia – has been reported when these natural foods are taken in combination with some conventional diabetes medications. Always be aware of the risk.

Key point: Enjoy okra and karela (bitter melon) in your newly varied diet. They may help to lower blood glucose and cholesterol a little, but you probably wouldn't want to eat them daily.

The goji berry – an example of a small superfood

The goji berry is a typical 'small' superfood that has been used for many years in traditional Chinese medicine, where it is added to herbal soups. We've seen that the large avocado doesn't contain sufficient amounts of any macronutrient (fat, carbohydrate or protein) to make any difference – unless you are an addict. The 'small' superfoods (usually berries) would therefore need to be consumed by the kilo if they were to have any chance of doing the same as olive oil. In addition, like the intriguing okra and karela, they may contain specific drug-like agents that help blood glucose, blood pressure, cholesterol or something else that's important to outcomes in diabetes. Below is a list of claims for the benefits of goji berries. Most small superfoods have a remarkably similar list of supposedly extraordinary therapeutic properties:

- high levels of antioxidants

- improve immune function and fight cancer
- promote healthy skin
- protect eye health
- help stabilise blood sugar
- detoxify the liver
- keep your energy and mood up
- boost fertility.

Antioxidants usually come at the top of the list. Most fruits and vegetables contain these fascinating substances. Test-tube experiments and studies in animals often show that antioxidants improve levels of anti-inflammatory compounds in the blood and tissues, but nobody has ever been able to find specific and measurable health benefits (other than the known benefits of a high-vegetable diet, such as the Mediterranean diet). Some of the other claims, for example improving immune function, fighting cancer and boosting fertility, are false, and a drug company claiming the same when there was no watertight evidence for a conventional drug would find themselves in court and billions out of pocket.

But like many of these foods, goji berries are interesting. There are warnings about interactions between goji berries and warfarin (a blood-thinner/anticoagulant), and some medications used in diabetes (sulfonylureas, for example, gliclazide), or for treating blood pressure. In the quantities most people will eat the berries it's unlikely they will have any serious side-effects, but it does remind us that like many other plants they contain bioactive chemicals. They haven't been identified yet. So yes to goji berries: a sprinkle over the porridge is tasty and pretty, but superfood – no.

Other berry superfoods

I won't repeat the claims for blueberries, acai, mulberries, chokeberries, maqui and countless other exotic 'superfood' berries because there are only minor variations on the goji list They have no specific actions in Type 2 diabetes, and are small and so expensive that they're only ever eaten in tiny quantities, so can have no benefits other than a fraction of any of your fruit and veg portions a day. But there'll never be any shortage of new rare berries enthusiastically endorsed as the next amazing superfood.

Key point: Antioxidants in berries and other foods are insufficient to deal with the body's oxidative stress.

Herb and spice 'superfoods'

There is a great deal of medical interest here, because herbs and spices often contain high concentrations of biologically active substances, and they are therefore of great interest to the drug industry. In addition, like the vegetables we've just discussed, they have found their way into traditional treatments around the world. Some have been studied in clinical trials in diabetes, usually to explore their effects on blood glucose levels, but only in small numbers of people, so it's very difficult to spot whether there is a genuine effect. Let's discuss two that have achieved superfood status – cinnamon and turmeric – and have been more widely investigated as nutraceuticals.

Cinnamon

Cinnamon hit the headlines in the mid-2000s and rapidly established itself as one of the earliest specific superfoods for reducing blood glucose levels in Type 2 diabetes. Since then, it's sunk in the popularity stakes, but studies still surface occasionally. The clinical trials highlight problems with studies of all plant derivatives. First, because many plants exist in different species and varieties it's very difficult to standardise the preparations used in a clinical trial. We say 'cinnamon', but there are four slightly different species used as spices in different parts of the world. *Cinnamomum cassia* (the main import into the USA) seems to be more effective in lowering blood glucose than the Sri Lankan forms – *Cinnamomum verum* or *Cinnamomum zeylanicum*. Botanical details apart, it's clear that 'cinnamon' powder or extract may be a variable mixture of different plants. So, in addition to all the other reasons why clinical trial results vary, in this case the medically active substance being tested may not even be the same. Second, as well as the variation in the plants themselves, there is no agreement on the best dose, and different studies have asked participants to take doses that range between 1 g and 5 g a day. You see the problems. Finally, because cinnamon is widely available and cheap, major pharmaceutical companies are not interested in producing standardised products which would be needed for reliable studies. (Recall that drugs need to undergo clinical trials in thousands of patients to observe any meaningful effects and the largest trials of herbs and spices have only included about 100 people.)

The general view is that any variety of cinnamon has no meaningful effects on either fasting blood glucose levels or glucose levels after meals, and no studies have shown an improvement in long-term glucose levels (that is, a reduction in HbA_{1c}). The highly authoritative USA National Center for Complementary and Integrative Health (see References, page 220) doesn't recognise cinnamon for the treatment or prevention of diabetes. So, let's enjoy it as ... cinnamon (but sadly not in the form of a very high-sugar iced bun).

Turmeric (curcumin)

Turmeric is a yellow spice widely used across south and south-east Asia as a curry spice and natural food colourant, and also in traditional medicine. Its rebirth as a potential treatment for diabetes occurred in the early 2000s. Its active ingredient is curcumin, a relatively simple chemical isolated nearly 200 years ago. It has multiple interesting effects on biochemical pathways that may be relevant in Type 2 diabetes (and in cancer and neurodegenerative diseases), but although there are many studies in test-tubes and animals, there are no meaningful clinical trial results in any of these conditions. It is quite difficult to understand how it has become so spectacularly popular, even in the highly commercialised and competitive world of superfoods.

Other spices and herbs

The list of spices and herbs supposedly effective in reducing blood glucose in Type 2 diabetes is huge, and includes:
- aloe
- cloves
- curry leaves
- fenugreek
- garlic
- ginger
- oregano.

None is supported by any clinical trial results that demonstrate useful blood glucose lowering properties, but many of them add wonderfully to the taste of food (and when used properly can reduce the need for seasoning with salt). Use and eat them all, and if clinical trial results do emerge that confirm some form of benefit, then we can always convince ourselves that that we were taking at least some of the right treatment all along. Putting all your therapeutically hopeful eggs in the fenugreek basket, however, doesn't seem sound.

Key point: In spite of promising chemistry, no herbs or spices have been shown to meaningfully and consistently reduce blood glucose levels.

Other nutraceuticals

Finally, let's turn to a varied group of supplements and minerals thought for many years to be useful in Type 2. Some have positive clinical trial results, but none has been approved because – as with the foods discussed earlier – trials haven't been performed in sufficient numbers of patients, the doses aren't standardised, and the results of small preliminary studies have not been consistent. I'll choose a few that people with Type 2 have mentioned to me recently.

Vinegar

Vinegar – specifically apple-cider vinegar – is often taken to reduce blood glucose levels. Does it? Probably yes, but only slightly. There have been some reasonable studies in non-diabetic people and Type 2s. How does it work? Probably through the acetic acid in vinegar reducing the conversion of carbohydrate to glucose, especially if the carbohydrate is high on the glycaemic index. Vinegar therefore lowers glucose levels only during and after meals – not overnight. A clever experiment showed that it's the acid that matters, not specifically the acetic acid found in vinegar, because sodium acetate, a salt that isn't itself an acid, has no blood glucose-lowering effect. The trials have been very short – a few days – so any effect on longer-term blood glucose measurements isn't known, but it looks as if it could reduce blood glucose levels after a meal by about 20% (for example, from 12 to 10 mmol/l) and if this was a consistent effect it could be meaningful. One trial used two teaspoons three times a day during each meal. Because all vinegar contains acetic acid, there's no need to buy expensive apple-cider vinegar: any vinegar will do. If you're going to try vinegar, make sure you don't take tablets that claim to be vinegar – they don't always contain what they say, and there's one report of 'vinegar' tablets causing ulceration of the oesophagus.

> **Key point:** A couple of teaspoons of vinegar with food might help reduce peak blood glucose levels after meals containing high GI carbohydrates.

Resveratrol

Resveratrol is found in grape skins. It's undoubtedly a very powerful chemical, and in the laboratory has some anti-cancer action, though there are no clinical studies. It's widely touted as a supplement for Type 2 diabetes. In 2016 a trial in Type 2s found that it did not help insulin resistance or liver fat (features of the metabolic syndrome, Chapter 3). There are no studies on blood glucose levels, but I'd be surprised if it turned out to have any useful effects.

Trace elements: chromium, vanadium and selenium

We need these three fascinating metals in tiny ('trace') amounts in the diet. An atom of each sits at the middle of complicated biological substances, for example enzymes, which help chemical reactions to continue. Deficiency of any of these can occur, but extremely rarely, because such small amounts are needed (for example, in one study men, though not women, were found already to be taking more than the recommended amount of chromium).

Chromium and vanadium are needed for metabolising carbohydrate, fat and protein, and about 20 years ago vanadium salts (vanadate) were researched in the hope they would help blood glucose levels in diabetes. The chromium story goes back even further – it was identified as a 'glucose tolerance factor' back in the 1950s. Chromium is naturally found in some foods, especially meat, wholegrain products, broccoli and red wine. There have been several investigations of chromium salts (usually chromium picolate) in small numbers of people with Type 2 diabetes. The bottom line is that chromium supplements have almost no effect on blood glucose levels. Cholesterol levels don't fall, and chromium doesn't help weight loss either.

Interestingly, there is one specific food that seems to have high chromium levels – brewer's yeast. You can get brewer's yeast tablets in any health food store, and yeast extract – Marmite in the UK, Vegemite in Australia – is mostly brewer's yeast. So, although there's no point in eating Marmite to help blood glucose levels or boost your chromium intake, eat it if you like it. In 2017 researchers found that some indicators of brain activity improved after Marmite, but not after peanut butter, and its effect on an important brain neurotransmitter (GABA) may be the reason. But not all countries think Marmite is great. For a long time, Denmark didn't allow sales of vitamin-foods such as Marmite, but in 2014 gave up and Danes can now eat it. Medically nothing has been proved, but no harm if you love it. This is the kind of discussion we should be having about most 'superfoods': if they are relatively low-carbohydrate and mesh nicely with the Mediterranean diet then they may be a tasty addition to meals. But individually none of them will save our lives.

Vitamins

Remember mega-dose vitamin C in the 1970s and '80s? Vitamins are the permanent superfoods: they never go away, and each of them hits the headlines for a while. About 10 years ago the vitamin D bandwagon started rolling. Vitamin D had always been on the medical radar because it's so important for maintaining bone strength. The ultraviolet part of the spectrum of sunlight is needed to convert cholesterol (yes, cholesterol) to vitamin D in the skin, so it's not surprising that people in northern countries are often low in vitamin D, especially in the winter. But we had no idea that so many people didn't have *any* detectable blood vitamin D. The story about the 'sunlight vitamin' exploded. Studies emerged every week linking vitamin D to countless conditions, especially the metabolic syndrome, hypertension and Type 2 diabetes. Then came the results of clinical studies in these areas – and, frustratingly, there was no benefit. We don't hear so much about vitamin D these days, and it won't help any aspect of your Type 2 (glucose, blood pressure, cholesterol).

The other main vitamins, A, the B group, C and E, all have important functions within different organs, but the body controls very carefully the amounts it retains (just as it does with trace elements), presumably because in excess they may be toxic. Type 2 patients with symptoms of numbness, pins and needles or pain in the feet and legs caused by peripheral neuropathy are often given B group vitamins, though there was never any evidence they helped. Doctors seem to love giving vitamins as much as patients love taking them. But there are warnings: in the mid-90s there was a huge trial of 'antioxidant' vitamins E and A taken separately or together in smokers who were therefore at risk of lung cancer. There was no benefit – but there was a higher overall death rate in the group taking a precursor of vitamin A (beta-carotene). Standard multivitamin preparations are probably harmless (and a huge clinical trial in Type 2 is currently in progress – see below), but I'd avoid high doses of individual vitamins.

Key point: If you have a good mixed diet, vitamin and mineral supplements aren't needed, and we still don't know whether multivitamins carry any health benefits.

Cocoa

Let's end the chapter on a positive note, and could there be anything more positive than the potential health benefits of chocolate? Cocoa beans, from which chocolate is made, contain high levels of biologically active flavanols. One of the main flavanols in cocoa is theobromine, derived from the botanical name for the cocoa tree,

Theobroma – Greek for 'food of the Gods'. We've heard about biologically active compounds in spices and herbs. They haven't fulfilled their biological promise in outcomes that are relevant to people, so is there anything different about cocoa flavanols? There may well be, because they don't act on a specific biochemical pathway, but are general and powerful relaxants of blood vessels, and there are many good-quality small studies showing that they increase the pliability and elasticity of arteries. Since arterial disease is partly due to stiff arteries, and arterial disease is the underlying problem in most of the complications of diabetes, flavanoids may help reduce heart attacks and strokes.

The National Institute of Health in the USA was sufficiently impressed by the potential for cocoa flavanols to improve vascular health that it funded a huge clinical trial (the Cocoa Supplement and Multivitamin Outcomes Study, COSMOS for short). It will enrol 18,000 people over 60. Half will take a standardised preparation of 600 mg cocoa flavanols twice a day for five years, the remainder a placebo (dummy) capsule. At the same time, subjects will take either a multivitamin tablet or a placebo. Vascular events, especially heart attacks and strokes, will be carefully documented as the primary outcome, but the trial is sufficiently powerful that it can also track other important outcomes – for example, cancer. It isn't specifically a trial in people with diabetes, though its large size means that many diabetic people will be included, and we know from other drug studies that any benefits in non-diabetic people are at least matched in people with diabetes. It should report toward the end of 2020 (and it will also help us decide whether it's worthwhile continuing our multivitamin pill-popping habit).

The flavanoid content of chocolate varies widely and you can't predict it from the stated percentage of cocoa solids (though milk chocolate and those with low cocoa levels will be higher in sugar, milk and calories). It looks as if you'd need to eat several ounces a day of dark chocolate (70% cocoa or higher) to even approach the flavanoid content of the capsules in COSMOS, and that would pile on your weight. But, as we've seen in several instances already, there are certain foods – including chocolate – that you can enjoyably include more frequently in your diet and that may eventually turn out to have health benefits in the long term.

Summary

Superfoods and nutraceuticals are always in the headlines. They contain a fascinating world of potential valuable substances, but none has been adequately investigated for its effects on diabetes – either short term on blood glucose levels or long term on the complications of diabetes. A few (for example okra and kerala) could usefully be incorporated into a healthy diet, but we should be eating lots of green veg anyway. Vinegar has a simple chemical effect that may reduce glucose levels after meals. Vitamins and minerals don't help diabetes. The COSMOS trial will tell us whether medicinal use of chocolate with or without multivitamins can improve vascular outcomes.

Chapter 7

Keeping your medication to a minimum

Key points

- Many Type 2s would like to reduce the amount of medication they take for blood glucose, blood pressure and cholesterol.
- Changes to diet can make meaningful differences – but the changes you need aren't always obvious. Fortunately there's clinical trial evidence to guide us.
- For blood glucose, losing weight and eating less, especially carbohydrates, allows many people to reduce their diabetes medication, and to take lower insulin doses.
- For blood pressure, reduce salt intake as much as possible, and keep alcohol to less than 14 units a week. Exercise may help.
- For cholesterol, a portfolio of specific foods e.g. plant-derived sterols (spreads or drinks), soy, okra, and nuts (also contained in the low-carbohydrate/Mediterranean diets) may have an effect. However, any effect is likely to be small in comparison with a statin.

Over-medication in diabetes

People with Type 2 diabetes often end up taking many different medicines, and understandably are unhappy about it. First, they are concerned about side-effects; second, every time they take medication it's a reminder of their Type 2 diabetes; third, the practicalities of getting enough supplies of medication are sometimes a hassle (renewing prescriptions, running out of medication, how to cope with long holidays – I needn't go on); and finally, people with newly diagnosed Type 2 know friends and relatives who have ended up on increasing amounts of medication over the years.

Fortunately, we don't need to be quite so concerned now about serious side-effects as a result of the regrettable history of Avandia (rosiglitazone), a drug introduced in the late 1990s. It reduced blood glucose levels effectively, but in long-term follow-up was linked with increased rates of heart attacks, bone fractures and anaemia. The USA Federal Drug Administration responded by requiring all new diabetes drugs to have long-term safety trials, focusing specifically on cardiovascular risks – that is, heart attacks and strokes. But these studies only need to start once the drug has been licensed for use, and they run for two to four years, so there is still a period after the introduction of drugs and before the final safety trials have reported during which there is a risk of new serious and previously unknown side-effects. We can be confident that all the new major groups of diabetes drugs have been through these trials (and semaglutide, a drug introduced in 2018, may have set a good example for the future: its cardiovascular safety trials were completed before the drug was launched, an extra reassurance). But no clinical trial, however huge and well conducted, can completely exclude the possibility of very long-term side effects, chief of which, of course, is cancer. Even with these new safety requirements successfully implemented, we must remain vigilant for side-effects that occur in individuals.

Key point: Regulations now make it more unlikely there will be serious unexpected side-effects from new drugs.

The frustration experienced by many people, especially when recently diagnosed, is that they feel they aren't given the time, encouragement or education to help improve their diabetes without the help of medication, and that it's a case of a brief introduction to lifestyle, followed in short order by a prescription for one or more tablets. They have an important point, though this scenario may be less common in places where all newly diagnosed people are encouraged to take part in a formal education programme (e.g. 'DESMOND' in the UK), and where people with diabetes have regular medication reviews, either with their diabetes team or, increasingly, by specialist pharmacists. A key question during these reviews is, or should be: is *every* item on a prescription list *really* necessary?

When medication is useful

Despite these concerns, medication is valuable when used with care and consideration, with due regard for individuals and their concerns, and their medical and social circumstances. Also, although medication is only very rarely immediately life-saving in the context of Type 2 diabetes, it can surprisingly quickly reduce the risks of major complications. For example, if blood pressure is found to be very high (systolic pressure more than 160 mm), prompt treatment with two different medications started at the same time reduced the risk of a stroke or heart attack over the next one to two years. Most doctors would use the medication approach rather than the slower and more unpredictable benefits of lifestyle intervention for initial treatment of very high blood pressure. The same goes for patients whose diabetes presents with serious symptoms due to very high glucose levels (see Chapter 2). Tablets, sometimes even insulin, are needed so that people can rapidly get on with their lives, though once the emergency is over, these emergency drug treatments can often be reduced when lifestyle interventions have started working. But where there is no such urgency, we should aim to start with minimum medication and maximum lifestyle intervention.

My prescription list seems to grow longer and longer ...

Nevertheless, over the years many people do tend to become burdened with more and more medication. Understandably, this doesn't do wonders for self-worth and can undermine motivation to self-manage. This is particularly the case for drugs to treat blood glucose levels, where progressive addition of tablets and injected treatments is a real concern.

During the 2000s, a major clinical trial (the ACCORD study) in people with about 10 years' diabetes attempted to keep blood glucose levels super-low (between 5 and 7 mmol/l) in order to find out whether this reduced the risk of heart attacks and strokes (it barely had any effect, as it happens – see Chapter 5). At the end of the trial, which lasted just over three years, the intensively treated group was taking on average just over three drugs for blood glucose, while the less-intensively treated group was taking two drugs. And these were just the blood glucose-lowering ones. In the same study, but this time focusing on blood pressure control, most people allocated to a very low blood pressure target were taking three drugs, and nearly one in five were taking five. So, to control blood pressure and blood glucose levels, admittedly to very low values which didn't help much to reduce long-term complications, many Type 2s might be taking five or six medications, and that's without a statin for cholesterol-lowering and aspirin for blood thinning (plus any other medications for non-diabetes problems). This could mean eight or more different drugs – a common scenario.

> **Key point:** Type 2s often end up taking many drugs. Although it's unlikely you will be able to ditch all medication, healthcare professionals and patients can work closely together to minimise the burden.

Guidelines for treatment usually focus on medication

Doctors often don't help the situation, though it's not entirely their fault. Every so often a group of experts issues 'guidelines' that – usually – urge us to aim for progressively lower blood glucose, blood pressure and cholesterol levels, and encourage us to use more complicated combinations of drugs, including newly introduced medications, to help achieve these lower targets. At the same time, other organisations tell doctors they aren't sufficiently 'proactive' and, even worse, they are accused of 'therapeutic inertia', which is medical-speak for doctors who don't act quickly enough to prescribe additional drugs to achieve the targets. Finally, once they've become more proactive and overcome their therapeutic inertia, they're encouraged to be 'aggressive' in their use of drug treatment. I don't much like the terms 'proactive' and 'therapeutic inertia', but 'aggressive treatment' seems to me a really unfortunate phrase in a supposedly caring profession. Of course, there's no implication of physical violence (though if I were a patient and overheard a reference to 'aggressive treatment' I might get a little anxious), but the implication is that at the very first sign of blood glucose levels rising, more and more medication needs adding – and as soon as possible. On rare occasions this may be the right thing to do – for example, where blood glucose levels are so high that a hospital admission is looming. This scenario was mentioned at the beginning of the chapter. But apart from emergencies, this approach is almost never needed, and when it is used quite often causes unnecessary anxiety in people who have been told they urgently need treatment.

Let's think about an approach that starts putting you more in control, so you can present information to your medical team that will convince them that, at the very least, you don't need *more* medication – and in fact may be in a good position to start reducing it. We will look in turn at each of the three main areas of Type 2 medication – blood glucose control, hypertension and cholesterol reduction, and examine what you can do in each case.

Blood glucose: will I always need some medication?

Newly diagnosed Type 2s often ask whether they will always need some medication for blood glucose control, and the answer is: no, they may not – for the reasons outlined in earlier chapters. Type 2 is potentially reversible, especially in the first five or so years after diagnosis, and one of the criteria to judge whether diabetes has been reversed is that blood glucose comes under control without the need for medication. There is also a small but interesting group of Type 2 people who have never needed medication and probably never will. They may have a form of diabetes that for some reason progresses ultra-slowly, but it's often because, right from the start, they were determined to minimise their tablet intake, and took the decision to substantially and permanently cut their calorie intake.

While most people are not in this fortunate situation, many can reduce their blood glucose-lowering medication, even if they can't completely ditch it altogether. The dietary approach is discussed in Chapter 5, and everyone can start their own diet experiment – for example, by trying to reduce their food intake by about 400 kcal/day while continuing to take their usual medication. This should result in fasting blood glucose levels falling substantially, perhaps by 2 or 3 mmol/l, and once this has happened, then your practice nurse or GP will be much happier to support a gradual reduction in medication. But the whole thing is a complex business that needs to be done carefully and slowly, reducing one medication at a time, while, of course, maintaining your calorie reduction.

Metformin forever?

One glucose-lowering medication widely considered to be a must for nearly all people with Type 2 is metformin. It was probably the medication you first started, and it's going to be the one that doctors will be most reluctant to let go. It is, in fairness, one of the oldest and most effective drugs (its active ingredient is derived from a plant extract – see Chapter 6, page 82), and the one that has never been shown to have any long-term adverse effects. In fact, a few years ago it was also thought to protect against some forms of cancers, but that enthusiasm has waned while we wait for the outcomes of large clinical trials. It doesn't usually cause hypoglycaemia (low blood sugar levels), though this can happen in some people if they're trying really hard with diet. Although metformin was supposed to cause significant weight loss, it's more accurate to say that it minimises weight gain. But these two properties – lack of hypoglycaemia and not causing weight gain – are two definite points.

In one trial, the United Kingdom Prospective Diabetes Study (UKPDS) (see References, page 214), metformin in overweight Type 2s showed some benefit in reducing the risks of heart attack. Ever since then, it has been widely thought that metformin has beneficial effects on the heart, independent of its blood glucose-lowering effect (and in 2015 someone even touted it as an anti-ageing drug that could increase life-expectancy to 120). In fact, no modern trials have confirmed the UKPDS finding, so although metformin is a safe and valuable drug for reducing blood glucose levels, as far as we know there are no additional advantages in taking it. Several clinical trials are in progress, investigating the effects of metformin on brain ageing and cardiovascular disease.

You may have some difficulty in persuading most doctors to let you off the metformin hook, as many still believe it has 'special' qualities. If you're taking metformin you could regard it as the only medication you need to continue in the long term. However, that is much better than taking an additional two or three drugs, with the prospect of another one being suggested every few years. But to get down to taking metformin alone often requires a good deal of determination, and nearly always major and permanent weight loss.

Sulfonylureas

The sulfonylureas (in the UK gliclazide is the most widely prescribed of this group of drugs) haven't had such a great press for a long time. There are no reports of major long-term side-effects but because they prod the pancreas into producing more insulin, and thereby reduce blood glucose levels, they can cause hypoglycaemia, particularly in people taking unaccustomed exercise or who miss meals. In addition, in the UKPDS, Type 2s taking older sulfonylureas that are no longer used gained weight and many people notice they stimulate the appetite. On the list of drugs that can be replaced by serious attention to weight loss, sulfonylureas are near the top. But they are quite powerful drugs for reducing blood glucose levels (they are often used at the time of diagnosis if blood glucose levels are very high), so after you and your diabetes team have decided to gradually decrease the dose of gliclazide, you need to maintain your enthusiasm for dieting and weight loss.

If you have successfully minimised or stopped a medication such as gliclazide by determined focusing on weight loss and diet, you are likely to want to go on and repeat the success story with other medications. But aiming to stop all your blood glucose medication for ever is very tough. The reality should be to minimise medication. As they say, the perfect must never be the enemy of the good. Nevertheless, whenever an additional medication is suggested, always consider whether it's really necessary, if the simpler solution might be reducing your calorie intake.

Doctors are very reluctant to admit that, right from the start, some medications don't work very well in some people. In addition, for a variety of reasons, all medications have a failure rate over time. Even metformin may become less effective with time, and the sulfonylureas are notable for their quite high rate of failure. In addition, there are some drugs which just aren't as effective as others in reducing blood glucose levels, even when they're working perfectly. The group of drugs whose names end in '-gliptin' (for example, sitagliptin, saxagliptin, vildagliptin) are generally weaker than other medications, so if you are taking one of these it could be relatively easy to discontinue it with additional attention to weight loss and carbohydrate intake.

> **Key point:** Sulfonylureas (for example, gliclazide) are the drugs most likely to cause hypoglycaemia, and they tend to increase weight and appetite. They would be a good focus in any medication-reducing programme.

Insulin

Insulin is the one medication that people most dislike taking, but unfortunately it is by far the most difficult to reduce or discontinue through weight loss, and any attempts at changing doses must always be done with the support of your medical team. Although compared with 20 years ago I think a smaller proportion of Type 2s now take insulin, the numbers are still very high, around 25–30%. In the past, most insulin-treated Type 2s took just insulin, but now it's usually combined with other medication, so perhaps they are taking fewer injections each day, a statistic that's probably not of much consolation to individuals using insulin. It's depressing that there are no studies on how to safely reduce insulin doses, or how successful it is: both these important omissions contribute to the understandable concern of patients that insulin treatment in Type 2 is always life long. However, it's well known that people whose diabetes is effectively 'cured' by bariatric surgery generally no longer need insulin after the operation, so it's important to recognise that the majority of insulin-taking Type 2 people are not 'insulin dependent'. Insulin is similar to the sulfonylureas, only more so: it tends to increase weight and appetite, and there is an even higher risk of hypoglycaemia. Type 2s who take insulin are highly aware of all these risks, and understandably it makes them even more keen to reduce their doses.

You'll first need agreement and support from your diabetes team. Abruptly discontinuing insulin, or reducing it by large amounts (for example, halving the dose) can result in rocketing blood glucose levels, and some hazard. There are many different kinds of insulin, and you would need a specific plan for the particular type and doses of insulin(s) you take. But we can use our new insight into Type 2 diabetes to make some educated judgements.

Remember the basic problem in Type 2 is the inability of the liver to control blood glucose levels overnight. That's why most people starting insulin begin with a bedtime dose of long-acting insulin that helps control high fasting glucose levels first thing in the morning. In the UK, the most frequently used long-acting insulins are Lantus and Levemir. There's also Abasaglar, Toujeo and Tresiba. The long-acting insulin is going to be the most difficult to reduce unless you lose the kind of weight seen in the Newcastle study (see Chapter 4, and page 213). In truth, most people taking one dose of long-acting insulin a day (usually at bedtime, but sometimes in the morning) don't mind injecting it, at least from the practical point of view of taking an injection.

But you can start making inroads if you are taking faster-acting or mixed insulin before one or more meals. A list of mealtime insulin preparations in common use in Type 2 diabetes in the UK is shown below.

Mealtime insulins used in the UK

Fast-acting 'analogue' insulins, usually taken before each meal:

- NovoRapid (aspart)
- Humalog (lispro)
- Apidra (glulisine)

Biphasic insulins (mixed short- and medium-acting) usually taken twice-daily before breakfast and the evening meal, but sometimes three times daily (additional dose before lunch):

- NovoMix 30
- Humulin M3
- Humalog Mix25
- Humalog Mix50

Mixed short-acting and long-acting:

- Ryzodeg

Mealtime insulin limits the rise in blood glucose after eating that is mostly caused by the amount of carbohydrate you take. Regularly limit your carbohydrate intake and you are likely to need less insulin at mealtimes. But again, this needs careful discussion with your diabetes team, who will probably suggest you measure blood glucose levels even more frequently after meals before and during any dose reduction.

I'll make one general point about different insulin preparations. In Type 2 diabetes there's almost no difference between one long-acting insulin and another. The same goes for short-acting mealtime insulins, and the mixed (biphasic) insulins. Manufacturers of new insulin preparations are understandably keen to promote small differences in the way these insulins act, and differences in the risk of hypoglycaemia. The way the insulin is used, and the engagement of the person using insulin, are both much more important than tiny differences seen in clinical trials, and we know this from studies over the years in younger people with Type 1 diabetes. Your current insulin is very likely to be fine. Only very rarely is there any need to change one insulin for another that acts in broadly the same way, and most importantly you are in control of your insulin, not vice versa.

> **Key point:** Don't suddenly discontinue or radically reduce the dose of any medication, especially insulin. Slow, gradual decreases tied in with strict dietary control, especially of carbohydrates, is the approach that's most likely to be successful.

Blood pressure

People with diabetes are less concerned about taking several different treatments to control blood pressure than for blood glucose. There are several reasons for this. Blood pressure doesn't have the same tendency as blood glucose to rise over the years, so you are less likely to be asked to take additional blood pressure medication. While blood pressure varies a little through the day (it's usually highest in the early morning and lowest in the middle of the night), it doesn't show the same dramatic swings as blood glucose, and doesn't need to be measured nearly as often. Finally, all medications for blood pressure control have been around for ages (the last major group of drugs was introduced nearly 20 years ago), so there's fortunately nothing new on the side-effect front that we haven't been aware of for a long time. You won't see headlines about either magic new drug treatments for blood pressure or shock-horror stuff about side-effects of older treatments (compare the seemingly never-ending statin saga; see Chapter 10). In short, blood pressure doesn't figure as prominently as blood glucose in the lives of people with Type 2, and the risk is that we can consider it to be less important than glucose. But we need to rethink our priorities. Blood pressure control is extremely important in reducing nearly all complications of diabetes and some, for example stroke risk, respond much better to blood pressure than glucose control.

Can any non-drug intervention really help blood pressure and reduce the number of drugs you need to take? Yes. But the warning about blood glucose control applies even more to blood pressure. Never reduce or stop blood pressure medication yourself. Blood pressure can rise very quickly if medication doses are reduced or stopped completely without having a proper plan in place. Bear in mind again the strong relationship between high blood pressure levels and stroke risk.

Key point: Don't reduce or discontinue any of your blood pressure medicines until you have a discussion with your healthcare team.

Before discussing non-drug interventions in more detail, the simplest option to reduce your medication might seem like a bit of a cheat, but it makes a lot of sense. Can you combine two of your blood pressure medicines in one pill? There are lots of these combined preparations around, they are always logical combinations, and haven't been introduced just on a whim. (Combination blood glucose medications are also widely available, usually metformin together with another drug.) Some doctors are quite keen to help people combine medications in this way, because it helps the troublesome business of tablet numbers. Others, often of an older generation, were taught at medical school that these so-called 'fixed-dose combinations' were the product of the devil and ought to be banned from the face of the earth. I'm with the first group. Any reduction in tablet numbers is to be welcomed, and if doctors don't support the use of combined medication it shows we don't appreciate the burden of daily tablet taking.

> **Key point:** If you are taking several medications for blood pressure, discuss with your medical team or pharmacist if two of them are available in a combined preparation.

The lifestyle portfolio for blood pressure

As with blood glucose, you can safely experiment with lifestyle changes, because any further blood pressure reductions are likely to be of long-term value. Work through in detail the blood pressure portfolio described below, and measure your blood pressure about twice a week while continuing to take your usual medication. Write the results down, show them to your healthcare team, and discuss whether there is any room for reducing your blood pressure medication. As you'd expect, the nearer your systolic blood pressure is to target (130 to 140 mm) the easier it will be to substitute permanent lifestyle change for medication.

Diet: adopt the DASH approach

Many studies have looked at the impact of lifestyle measures on blood pressure, so at least we have a firm basis for recommending what is likely to work. Equally important, we have some idea of what doesn't work, and chief among these is – surprisingly – weight loss by itself. Since being overweight is associated with high blood pressure, you'd expect weight loss itself to lower blood pressure. It doesn't: we saw that 15 kg weight loss in the Newcastle study didn't reduce blood pressure, and even huge weight loss, as much as 40 kg after bariatric surgery, only has a small effect on blood pressure.

However, when weight loss and exercise are combined – for example, in the Look AHEAD study (see Chapter 5, page 58) – blood pressure does fall, and the reduction can be quite impressive, similar to the effect of drugs in the ACCORD study (see page 101). In general, lifestyle intervention is more successful in very overweight people with a BMI greater than 30, while drug treatment seems to be better in the less overweight.

The DASH diet for hypertension (DASH stands for 'Dietary Approaches to Stop Hypertension') is now 20 years old, but was way ahead of its time. It emphasised fruits and vegetables, low-fat dairy products and encouraged low saturated fats and total fats, though it was before the era of encouraging 'good' fats – for example, the monounsaturated oils of nuts and olive oil; these, as we have seen (in Chapter 5), were the focus of the PREDIMED approach. Nevertheless, it was dramatically successful and reduced systolic blood pressure by 11 mm in hypertensive people, which is the equivalent effect of at least one, and in some people two, medications.

Cut down your salt intake

Too much salt causes fluid retention and increases blood pressure. The link was established years ago; conversely, reducing salt intake reduces blood pressure in many people. (An unseemly scientific quarrel lasting decades has blunted the impact of this 'fact', and as I write this, a USA research scientist is advocating eating any amount of salt that you feel is right.) There are concerns that the false controversy over salt intake and cardiovascular disease risk is in some ways similar to the climate change 'debate'. We can never be 100% certain of the link, because we'll never be able to do the experiment comparing life expectancy in a group forced to eat a high-salt and another a low-salt diet, but for the majority of scientists and doctors, the evidence is pretty compelling: too much salt is bad for everyone, but especially for people with high blood pressure.

The recommendation is to eat less than the equivalent of one teaspoonful of salt a day (2.3 g), and if you're over 50 less than ½ teaspoonful (1.2 g). On average we eat *hugely* more than that. In a recent survey, most people take between 6 and 12 g a day – that is, between two and five times the recommended maximum. However, encouragingly, in the UK average daily salt intake fell from about 9.5 g a day in 2003 to 8 g in 2011 – still far too much, but heading in the right direction. This reduction itself may have been responsible for much of the reduction in strokes that occurred over the same period. In spite of nearly everyone claiming that they don't add salt to their meals, most people are aware that pre-prepared food contains most of the salt we eat. Vegetarian foods are no lower in salt than non-veg foods. Some examples:

Standard white bread	0.7 g per slice
Packet of salt and vinegar crisps	1 g
Shop-bought prawn sandwich	0.8 g
Pre-packed vegetarian sushi selection	1.1 g
3 chocolate digestive biscuits	0.6 g
Half a can of tomato soup	1.1 g
Two slices of bacon	0.3 g

The best safeguard against eating too much salt is to do as much of your own cooking as possible, and minimise shop-bought snacks and sandwiches. (And point out to the smug people who proudly state they never add salt to their meals that a generous pinch of salt is only about 0.3 g, while a packet of crisps contains three times that amount.)

Key point: Reducing your salt intake can make meaningful inroads into blood pressure, up to 10 mm lower, similar to the DASH diet, and the equivalent of one or two different blood pressure medications.

Keep the alcohol down

Until recently I wasn't aware that excess alcohol was associated with high blood pressure, but this is part of a recent reassessment of evidence on the impact of alcohol on general health. This takes into account the increased risk of cancer (including breast cancer), and possibly of Alzheimer-type dementia. In 2016 the recommended alcohol limit for both men and women was decreased to 14 units a week (for example, 7 pints of beer), compared with the previous guidance of 21 units or less for men, and 14 for women. On the more positive side, in Type 2 diabetes, moderate alcohol intake is linked to a lower risk of eye and kidney complications, but heavy alcohol drinking increases overall cardiovascular risk. Whether it is alcohol itself, or specifically red wine that is responsible for vascular benefits has never really been sorted out, because it's difficult to find populations who drink only beer, or only white or red wine.

Focusing on blood pressure in people with Type 2, $\frac{1}{3}$ of a bottle of red wine daily in women and about ½ bottle in men (3 to 5 units a day – well over the current recommended limit) had no impact on blood pressure or blood glucose levels. But the evidence on heavy alcohol intake is clear: it increases many risks, particularly strokes and heart attacks, and in very heavy alcohol users, a short period without alcohol reduced blood pressure by 8–13 mm, whether or not they were already hypertensive.

> **Key point:** Limiting alcohol intake, for example up to the current recommended limit (14 units a week), may reduce the risk of cardiovascular events and eye and kidney complications. Risks of many diseases increase rapidly above this level of drinking.

Exercise

Exercise doesn't reduce weight (see Chapter 8), but it can really help blood pressure. Three times a week intensive treadmill exercise can reduce blood pressure by about 10 mm, and the same frequency of resistance training (weights) may also help.

Complementary and alternative treatments

There is a long list of nutraceuticals that may help hypertension. Where they have been studied, each reduces systolic blood pressure by a small amount, around 2 mm, but combined they are likely to have a more marked effect. Note the overlap here with many of the components of the Mediterranean diet. One, cocoa, has been of interest for a long time, especially because it contains flavanoid chemicals that relax blood vessels and help blood pressure, and chocolate regularly emerges as a 'superfood' (see Chapter 6, page 95).

Nutraceuticals potentially helpful for hypertension include:

- flaxseed, folate, garlic
- soy protein, fish oils, olive oil
- flavanoids: tea (green tea probably has a bigger effect than black tea), grapes, cocoa
- high fibre.

Herbal suggestions include hawthorn and various traditional Chinese herbal medicine formulas. Meditation-based interventions, including Qi Gong and Tai Chi, reduce blood pressure in smaller controlled trials, but it seems as if regular exercise is the key factor here, not whether it is conventional or traditional. Biofeedback has been around for many years, but little positive support has emerged from clinical trials.

> **Key point:** To help reduce blood pressure: minimise salt, keep alcohol intake to less than 14 units a week, exercise, and do your best with the Mediterranean/DASH diet.

Cholesterol

Non-drug management of high cholesterol levels has been downgraded just as we encountered in hypertension. The reason is that statins are very safe, can reduce cholesterol levels by up to 50% (even more if combined with other medication) and, most important of all, reduce vascular risks by around 40% (see Chapter 10). Non-drug management of cholesterol can reduce blood levels – in trials quite substantially – but it's unlikely that dietary portfolios could either be maintained in the long term or significantly reduce heart attack and stroke risk. However, several foods and nutraceuticals used in trials not surprisingly also figure in the lower-carbohydrate and Mediterranean approaches we discussed in Chapter 5.

What are the best foods to lower cholesterol?

There is a link between high saturated fat diets and blood cholesterol, but it's a weak link. However, less red meat and processed meats is probably a good start – the latter also contain a lot of salt. Remember that very few foods contain cholesterol, and even when they do (for example, eggs) eating them doesn't translate into higher blood cholesterol, and can even boost protective/ good HDL levels. Zero-cholesterol foods won't help your blood cholesterol levels, and they're often packed with carbohydrates and sugars.

Plant sterols/stanols

Specific nutraceuticals can reduce cholesterol levels. The most powerful are the plant stanols/sterols added to margarines and drinks (e.g. Benecol, Flora ProActiv, and various supermarket own-brand products). The most effective daily intake is about 2 g, which is contained in two tablespoonsful of margarine or a small individual drink. They consistently reduce LDL cholesterol, the portion of circulating cholesterol which causes most damage to arteries, by about 13%. This isn't anywhere near the reduction needed in most Type 2s to get LDL to the recommended level of less than 3 mmol/l – around 30–50% – but it's significant, and a non-statin drug, ezetimibe, that has about the same effect, reduced coronary events in a major clinical trial by about 10%. But you need to take your drink or margarine in the right amount, and every day. I'd suggest the drinks rather than the spread: you'd need several slices of bread to accommodate the two large spoonfuls of margarine, and that might not be so good for the lower-carbohydrate approach. Ensure that any drinks are low-calorie.

Other foods that can help reduce cholesterol

Foods that actively reduce cholesterol levels are individually much less effective than the plant stanols/sterols. Each can reduce cholesterol by about 2%, which is too small to detect on routine blood tests, but taken together as a portfolio they are likely to be more effective, and perhaps boost the effect of the plant stanols supplement by a few percentage points. But regardless of their cholesterol-lowering effects, we encountered several of them in the lower-carbohydrate and Mediterranean diets. See Table 7.1.

Table 7.1 A portfolio approach to non-drug reductions in cholesterol levels.

Food/ nutraceutical	Recommended amount	Comments
Soy protein (soy milk, tofu, soy 'meat' products)	1½ ounces daily	Soy is an important high-protein food incorporated into south-east Asian cuisines. It's much more interesting and varied than soy 'milk'. Most of the clinical trials of soy protein haven't shown a reduction in cholesterol levels.
Soluble fibre	Around ¾ ounce daily	Barley, oats, aubergine, okra (see Chapter 6).
Nuts	Around 1½ ounces daily	In the PREDIMED study this intake was associated with a reduction in heart attacks.

Food/ nutraceutical	Recommended amount	Comments
Plant sterols	Margarine (2 tablespoons) or 1 yoghurt drink daily	
General advice		Vegetables, eggs, whole-grain cereal, low-fat dairy, fruit; reduce red meat and snacks.

Key point: A daily intake of 2 g of plant sterols/stanols (margarine, yoghurt drink) can reduce LDL cholesterol levels by about 13%. But you'll still need a statin.

What's realistic minimum medication for Type 2s?

A very small proportion of people need no medication at all for their diabetes. These fortunate people will be Type 2s with only slightly high blood glucose that can be managed with diet alone, and whose blood pressure and cholesterol levels are naturally at target. Interestingly, this profile is often seen in young people with Type 1 diabetes. Later-onset Type 1 diabetes in people is being diagnosed more frequently and perhaps up to 20% of older people thought to have Type 2 diabetes, because they were diagnosed in their 30s, 40s and 50, may actually have Type 1. They tend not to be too overweight, and like the younger Type 1s have life-long naturally low blood pressure and a nice cholesterol profile. Type 2 patients from China and other south-east Asian countries also have these characteristics.

But these are small numbers, and there are almost no Type 2s not taking any medication. Strenuous attempts to stick to your lifestyle portfolios may allow you to cut your medication back to the following. It still looks like a lot of tablets, but it's a lot less than eight or nine medications, which isn't uncommon:

- metformin
- one medication for blood pressure
- a statin
- low-dose aspirin in people who have had a stroke or heart attack.

And as we've seen, if there is a 'threat' to increase your medication, a determined and focused effort using the considerable evidence that we now have on lifestyle changes may well result in a postponement of another pill to pop every day.

Summary

If you pay detailed attention to your diet, weight loss and activity you should, with support from your healthcare team, be able to reduce the amount of medication you take. This will improve your numbers (glucose, blood pressure and possibly cholesterol) and, combined with a broader approach to your diet, for example the Mediterranean, is likely to reduce your risk of diabetic complications in the longer term. But don't reduce medication by yourself: always discuss it first with your diabetes team.

Chapter 8

Activity and exercise

Key points

- We'd all love to become super-fit sleek athletes, but if you have Type 2, then be reasonably happy with the beneficial effects of exercise on general fitness, vascular disease and blood glucose levels.
- Moderate and vigorous exercise reduces heart attack and stroke rates and eye and kidney complications.
- Regular exercise improves glucose levels a little.
- For those who can manage it, high-intensity exercise reduces glucose levels (e.g. four to six bouts of all-out sprinting or cycling for 30 seconds two or three times a week).
- Aerobic ('cardio') exercise and anaerobic exercise (resistance/weights) should both be part of a full exercise regimen. Resistance training reduces blood glucose levels and the amount of fat in fatty liver.
- Tech aids, for example pedometers, haven't lived up to their promise, and don't consistently increase activity levels.

Physical activity for people with Type 2

You'll know Oscar Wilde's famous views on exercise – 'whenever I feel the urge to exercise, I go and lie down'. The modern equivalent may be your response to seeing some lean young thing running down the street faster than the traffic and wearing the latest hi-vis sportswear while ensuring that all the more sedentary people are aware they are in the presence of someone who owns the latest and most expensive Fitbit. It's all a bit dispiriting for us middle-aged people. It's even more difficult when there are physical difficulties, such as back pain, leg problems and general aches and pains, and stresses such as a hectic life full of things that demand more immediate attention than exercise. In addition, it's well known that people with Type 2 – even if they are in generally good health – tend to have lower exercise tolerances than those without diabetes.

Physical activity (exercise is a more structured and focused form of physical activity) is surrounded by almost as many myths and uncritically accepted truths as diet. When we are told that exercise is 'good' for us, what does that actually mean? Most people accept that regular exercise generally makes us feel better, and that's usually attributed to the release of happy hormones such as endorphins, but in addition, in diabetes we'd like to gain more specific benefits from exercise. I'm going to look at some of the evidence for the impact of exercise on blood glucose levels, weight and diabetes complications. We'll start by comparing our individual activity against the World Health Organization's (WHO) recommended amount of exercise, adopted by many countries, including the UK.

The WHO recommendations on activity

Adults up to their mid-60s should do moderate-intensity exercise (we'll discuss what that means shortly) for at least 150 minutes a week, or 75 minutes of vigorous-intensity activity. The simple arithmetic works out at 20 minutes of moderate-intensity or just over 10 minutes of vigorous-intensity every day. That's quite a time commitment. The WHO goes on to say that for 'additional' health benefits the 150 minutes needs doubling to 300 minutes – that is, over 40 minutes a day. If you're 65 or older, the same recommendations apply, but in people with mobility problems, activity to improve balance and reduce the risk of falls should be done three times a week. Top of the list of benefits of regular activity relevant to Type 2s are improving muscle fitness and cardiac and respiratory (lung) fitness. Bone health and reducing the risk of falls and of hip or spine fractures also figure. We've already discussed activity and how it might reduce the risk of developing Type 2 diabetes (Chapter 3), but remember that the only study showing that exercise by itself (without additional weight loss) delayed the onset of Type 2 was in Chinese people with pre-diabetic glucose levels, so people of other ethnicities need both exercise and weight loss to achieve the same effect. The risk of some cancers (for example, bowel and breast) is reduced through exercise, but meaningful reductions in risk are only seen with 300 minutes or more a week.

Key point: The World Health Organization recommends 20 minutes a day of moderate intensity exercise or 10 minutes of vigorous intensity for promoting good general health.

These health benefits are not to be sniffed at, but we really need some hard evidence – if there is any – for long-term outcomes of exercise in people with diabetes. Fortunately there is some, though not as much as you might expect – from the ADVANCE study in the USA, which was designed to study heart attack and stroke rates over a five-year period. Participants were older people, average age 66, with about eight years of Type 2. Activity levels were classified as follows, so this gives us some idea of what is meant by mild, moderate and vigorous exertion:

- mild exercise: easy walking, bowling
- moderate exercise: fast walking, tennis, dancing
- vigorous exercise: jogging, vigorous swimming.

On average, the moderate or vigorous exercisers were doing over three hours (180 minutes) of activity a week, and therefore more than the WHO recommendation (150 minutes). There were no benefits if you did mild exercise, but all the important outcomes of diabetes were reduced by 15–20% in the two other groups: vascular events (heart attack and stroke), kidney and eye complications (see Chapter 11) and mortality rates. We don't have confirmation of this result in other studies, but it is a very striking finding in a huge number of people (around 11,000 took part in the study). The negative conclusion is that mild activity doesn't carry long-term benefits. We'll discuss this more, but the sad news is that gentle walking that doesn't make us even slightly short of breath or increase our pulse rate is not meaningful activity, at least when judged by diabetes outcomes.

Key point: In Type 2, moderate or vigorous activity for three hours a week reduces the risk of many of the complications of diabetes.

Levels of exercise

The WHO gives some additional examples of moderate and vigorous activities, and also introduces us to the MET (metabolic equivalent of a task), a number that represents the *intensity* of exercise, which is more important than just the duration. One MET is the amount of energy we expend when sitting quietly. Mild exercise – which, as we've seen, probably doesn't do much for our health – is defined as a MET value of less than 3 (that is, up to three times the energy we use when sitting). Moderate exercise has a MET value of between 3 and 6, and vigorous activity more than 6. Table 8.1 gives some examples, and Figure 8.1 shows a graphic of some of these forms of activity.

Table 8.1 Examples of different levels of activity and their MET values

Mild activity (less than 3 METs)	Moderate-intensity activity (3–6 METs)	Vigorous-intensity activity (more than 6 METs)
	Requires a moderate amount of effort, and noticeably increases your heart rate	Requires a lot of effort, with rapid and heavy breathing, and a major increase in heart rate
Emailing	Brisk walking	Running
Watching TV	Dancing	Walking or climbing briskly up a hill
Computer use	Gardening	Using cardiovascular (cv) equipment
Caring for adults	Housework and domestic chores	Aerobics
Music and performing activities	Active involvement in games and sports with children	Fast swimming
Shopping	Gentle cycling (under 10 mph)	Fast cycling (more than 10 mph)
	Home exercises	Martial arts
	Yoga, weight lifting, strength training	Roller-blading
	Walking pets	Competitive sports and games
	General building (e.g. painting)	Heavy shovelling
	Carrying or moving moderate loads (lighter than 3 stones)	Carrying or moving heavy loads (heavier than 3 stones)
	Sexual activity (you always wanted to know that)	

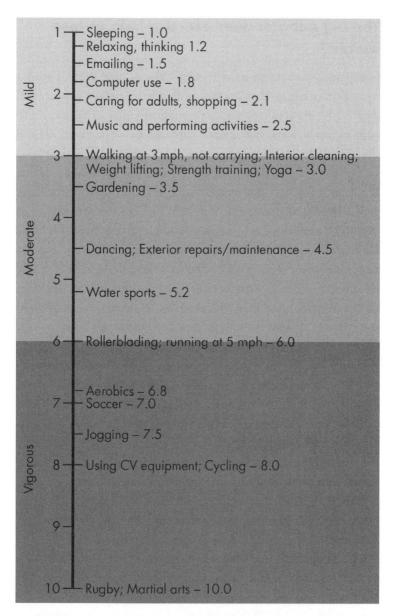

Figure 8.1: The intensity of some activities (METs). Intensity lower than 3 is considered mild, between 3 and 6 moderate and vigorous if METs are greater than 6. (Running at 7 mph is 11.5 and at 9 mph is 15.)

The big debate: does exercise help us lose weight?

Companies that tempt us with high-calorie, high-sugar, high-fat food always tell us that exercise will help us reduce weight, and that it isn't the fault of their tempting products. You may have your personal view, but science here can be of practical help in shedding light on the 'exercise vs. diet' debate. For example, if you expend 400 kcal of energy every day doing exercise, then it *should* result in the same weight loss as if you reduced your calorie intake by the same amount. Why don't we see the equivalence in real life? The reason, as usual, is not that science is wrong; it's that we're humans and not machines. Our bodies and metabolism are amazingly efficient: we rapidly extract nearly all the usable energy stored in food, and the muscles use that energy with an efficiency that man-made machines will probably never achieve. The food manufacturers omit to tell us that their products have a high energy density (that is, the number of calories in a single mouthful is large), and getting rid of that energy is very time consuming, no matter how intensively you exercise. Let's take 400 kcal as an example – see the box below(participants in the DiRECT low-carbohydrate study who reduced their calorie intake by 400 kcal lost about 5 kg – see Chapter 5).

Exercise required to burn up 400 kcal

What do 400 food calories look like? Usually: quick and easy. The average pre-prepared sandwich from any major outlet contains ... 400 kcal. Grabbed from the shelf and guzzled in about *four* minutes while dealing with emails. How long does it take to burn off those 400 exercise calories? It's nearly always: slow and difficult. Someone weighing about 12 stone (170 lb or 77 kg) would need to – wait for it:

- cycle for an *hour* at 10 mph
- do gardening for three *hours*

- jog for one *hour*
- play golf for three-and-a-half *hours*.

(Every day, remember.) No contest. In the perfect world we all choose the exercise option; in the real world we grab and guzzle the sandwich. Losing meaningful amounts of weight through exercise isn't much of an option for most of us.

Other estimates confirm this painful conclusion. For example, The American College of Sports Medicine estimates that to reduce your weight by between 5 and 10% (you will recall that 10% was achieved for a short time in Look AHEAD) you need to do between four and seven hours of moderate or vigorous aerobic exercise a week. The weekly recommended 150 minutes of moderate exercise will achieve, at best, about 2 or 3 kg weight loss, and many people will see no changes in their weight. Resistance training is not very effective for weight loss – though it is recommended for strengthening muscles as part of the WHO exercise regimen. Interestingly, resistance training lowers blood glucose levels (see below) and fatty liver responds well to it.

Let's look at a couple of other exercise-related theories:

- **Can exercise reduce the risk of regaining weight after dietary weight loss?** There are very few of us who haven't experienced a dispiriting regain in weight after working really hard at dieting. This is one area where a focus on exercise may be very helpful. To minimise the risk of gaining weight again you need about three hours (200 minutes) of moderate activity a week, which is substantially more than the WHO recommendation, but if you've been motivated sufficiently to lose weight in the first place, you may well be able to move to an enhanced exercise regimen without too much difficulty.
- **'Fit but fat': does it exist?** The 'fit but fat' slogan rolls off the tongue easily, but has the same problem as many

catchphrases: it oversimplifies. None of us is 'either' fit or fat: each individual has a unique combination of both fatness and fitness (fitness means 'cardiorespiratory fitness' – that is, how well the heart and lungs cope with activity). The conclusion from all the statistical to-ing and fro-ing (and you can imagine how much of that there's been) is no great surprise: whatever your weight, increased activity – along the WHO lines – reduces the risk of vascular events, and in people with diabetes, probably also reduces the risk of the more specific eye and kidney complications, as well as stimulating the liver to get rid of its fat. But there are competing factors here: the heavier you are the more likely you are to have Type 2, high blood pressure and abnormal cholesterol levels, all of which are risk factors for diabetes complications. If you have a high burden of risk factors, then you're likely to need *more* exercise to counterbalance their adverse effects.

The conclusion to take away from this research is: do your best both to lose weight and to increase your exercise levels. So, eat 400 kcal fewer each day and go all out for 20 minutes of moderate or heavier exercise a day.

Key point: If you exercise – moderate activity or heavier – for three hours a week after losing weight with diet, it should limit weight regain.

Exercise and blood glucose levels

Diabetic people who use insulin, especially Type 1s, notice that blood glucose levels can fall very rapidly, even after taking a gentle stroll, and Type 1 patients often tell me that if they do a blood test and find an unexpected high glucose level, 10–20 minutes of brisk walking will often do the trick and lower it. This rapid response is due to several different effects of insulin. If you have Type 2, but don't take insulin, can exercise lower blood glucose levels?

You might think we have a clear answer to this, but there are few large-scale trials, and the smaller ones use all manner of different exercise regimens, so it's difficult to draw firm conclusions. The general view is that regular aerobic exercise in Type 2 diabetes can modestly reduce HbA_{1c} levels, by around 0.5% (which is not to be sniffed at – some drugs aren't much more effective). But there's precious little evidence that even those who diligently take their 150 minutes' exercise a week see much benefit in blood glucose levels. This is disappointing but by now shouldn't come as much of a surprise; everyone with Type 2 is different and all respond differently, even to the same treatment. The wise approach is to take part in any regular form of exercise that you enjoy, try and boost it to the WHO recommended level each week, and recognise that it's likely to contribute – together with all the other parts of the diabetes lifestyle portfolio – to a long-term reduction in major complications, even though you may see no major changes in blood glucose levels. Perhaps there may be more subtle improvements: nearly three-quarters of a group of well-controlled Type 2 people in Denmark were able to reduce their diabetic medication in a trial of aerobic training sessions lasting 30–60 minutes every week for six weeks.

Technology and activity

Activity is now heavily linked with social media, apps and software, gadgets and the 'internet of things'. These all carry the wow factor of new technology (and 'eHealth'), and increase the 'glamour' aspects of exercise, but in spite of their popularity and the money we spend on them, there are very few studies of their long-term effectiveness. In addition, they can become associated with a degree of dogma that we're very familiar with from the world of diets. For example, the exercise equivalent of 'eggs are bad for you' (no they're not) could well be '10,000 steps a day are good for you' (not proven). Actually the 10,000 steps a day 'rule' seems to have emerged with the invention of the first pedometer in Japan around the time of the Tokyo Olympics in 1960. And why 10,000? Apparently 10,000 is a lucky number in several oriental cultures. So, there's *no* scientific or health basis for the 10,000 steps 'rule' as applied to individuals, but it chimes very nicely with cool pedometers and apps. Walking 10,000 steps is the equivalent of five miles a day – that is, at least an hour and a quarter of walking and nearly nine hours a week. Most of us find it difficult to reach the WHO recommendation of 150 minutes a week, so this is an unrealistic aim for nearly everyone, and recall from our previous discussion that *intensity* of exercise is as important as the amount; 10,000 steps of fast walking up and down hills isn't the same as 10,000 steps strolling gently round the shops.

Clinical trials of pedometers in non-athletes are mostly disappointing, in large part because we quickly get bored with gadgets. In a study of Fitbits in working people in Singapore, only about 10% were using them after a year. Encouraging participants to exercise by offering cash slightly increased their activity levels compared with those who weren't paid, but the effect lasted only as long as the money. Giving pedometers to first-year university students didn't increase their activity levels, and also had no effect on their psychological wellbeing. Using pedometers does not improve blood glucose control in Type 2 diabetes. A stylish device, even one that's linked to social media and route-planning is likely to remain just that – a stylish device.

However, integrating activity into our everyday life, especially in the workplace, carries more promise, and justifiably has recently become a fruitful field for research, as has the fascinating field of planning the urban and working environments to encourage ('nudge') us into increasing our level of day-to-day activity.

Key point: Aiming for an arbitrary (and high) number of steps a day is no substitute for thinking about the duration and intensity of your activity.

Activity at work

Most of us work sitting down. You're likely to spend about six and a half hours a day sitting, usually at a computer terminal (and much of the time getting stressed by it). Most doctors are no different. Some people have turned to gadgetry to try and boost their activity levels: a recent vogue is for standing desks. I suspect they'll be used about as long as the pedometers, and nobody has shown any major health benefits. But incorporating increased activity into your existing work schedule is more sound, and may carry some of the benefits for blood glucose control of intermittent high-intensity exercise (see below). For example, in a recent study in overweight Type 2 people, blood glucose levels fell for nearly 24 hours after exercising for three minutes every half hour during a simulated seven-hour working day. Aerobic exercise (walking) and simple resistance activities (half-squats, calf and knee raises) were equally effective. Fasting blood glucose levels the next day fell by 2 mmol/l: if this effect persisted, then there should be an effect on HbA_{1c} levels after about two to three months. We await confirmation, but practicable suggestions for further increasing activity at work include the following:

- stand to greet a visitor to your workspace
- walk to a colleague's desk rather than phoning, texting or emailing
- drink more water (nothing to do with the 'hydration' myth, but increased visits to the water cooler – and loo – help to break up sitting time)
- move your waste bin away from your desk, but walk to it, and don't use it to improve your target skills for waste paper

- don't eat lunch at your desk
- stand at the back of the room during presentations rather than sit down
- use your office stairs
- don't use lifts for journeys of less than two floors.

High-intensity exercise (HIT)

Over the past few years there's been a lot of interest in a new form of exercise: high-intensity activity. Examples include 30 seconds of sprinting at maximum speed or all-out cycling (stationary bike) for 30 seconds. In the classic studies, each activity was repeated four to six times separated by about four minutes of no exercise or relaxed activity. Careful studies in people with pre-diabetes or Type 2 show that muscles start working very efficiently after this form of exercise, and in particular take up more glucose from the circulation. Although the obvious effect is to reduce blood glucose levels, the really important effect is increasing the efficiency with which insulin operates. And it has a surprisingly quick effect: after six sessions spread over just two weeks muscle glucose uptake was already more effective.

Of course, not everyone can do this form of exercise, which may be more suitable for younger people or those who have had diabetes for a short time. It focuses on leg exercise (our largest muscles are in the legs), so that's another reason why it might not be suitable for people with arthritis or trouble with the peripheral nerves leading to neuropathy. But for people who can manage it, it's worthwhile, and is less time consuming than conventional aerobic exercise. In one study of cycling, four to six sessions spread over two weeks, each lasting 40–60 seconds had about the same effect on blood glucose levels as the same number of 30-second all-out cycling bursts. HIT seems also to benefit cardiac function and reduces liver fat in Type 2 people.

Summary

Moderate or intensive activity (that is three or more METs) for two and a half hours or more a week improves many aspects of general health and also reduces the risk of most of the complications of diabetes. Intermittent exercise at work may also turn out to have long-term benefits in the majority of us who are sedentary during the majority of the working day. Exercise itself doesn't consistently reduce blood glucose levels but probably improves other features of the metabolic syndrome – for example, hypertension fatty liver. Elaborate and conspicuous sportswear and technology haven't been shown to improve health.

Chapter 9

Looking after your heart and arteries

Key points

- Major heart attacks still occur more often in Type 2 people than in non-diabetic individuals, but they have become much less common over the past 20 years.
- Other arterial diseases in Type 2 (leading to strokes, amputations and kidney failure) have also decreased.
- However, smaller heart attacks which don't always cause symptoms and which can cumulatively weaken the heart muscle and cause heart failure are more common.
- Much the same is happening in strokes: major strokes resulting in severe disability are less common, but smaller events including transient ischaemic attacks (TIAs/mini-strokes) and 'lacunar' strokes deep in the brain are very common, and easy to spot on brain scans.
- Arterial disease in the legs is less frequent as well, in part because fewer people smoke.
- X-ray techniques to open up blocked arteries continue to improve, but long-term medication and lifestyle portfolios are needed to reduce the risk of arteries becoming blocked again.

Heart attacks and Type 2 diabetes in the past 20 years

A man is as old as his arteries and his interests. If he permits his economic, religious, or social arteries to harden, or loses

*interest in whatever concerns mankind ... he will need only
six feet of earth.*

Josephus Daniels (USA, 1862–1948)

One of the great diabetes experts of my generation is a serious
scientist and a humourous Scot called Miles Fisher. He has always
been interested in the impact of diabetes on the heart, and over
20 years ago he made the following observation, considered
provocative when he first stated it in 1996, but time has proven
him to be spot on:

*Diabetes is a state of premature cardiovascular death which
is associated with high blood glucose levels sustained over
a long time and may also be associated with blindness and
renal failure.*

He was telling us that the really important thing for people
with Type 2 diabetes is the risk of heart disease. He also went
on to say that this increased risk is *associated* with high blood
glucose levels sustained over a long period of time. He was –
note – not saying that the heart disease is *caused* by high blood
glucose levels: it is one of several contributory factors, chief
among them high blood pressure and LDL cholesterol. He then
went on to list two additional major and feared complications
of diabetes, blindness and renal failure, which are discussed in
Chapter 11, and which since 1996 have fortunately become
much less common, just like classical heart attacks.

Key point: High blood glucose levels contribute to heart
attacks and strokes in people with diabetes, but are not the
sole reason for these complications.

I took up my consultant post in 1995, a year before Miles made
his dramatic statement. And he was completely right: when I did

my general ward rounds, and passed by the coronary care unit, it was like doing the nightmare version of a diabetes outpatient clinic. 'Hi, Dr Levy, nice to see you.' 'What happened, Mrs Patel/ Mr Smith?' 'A heart attack.' Fast forward 20 years, and we'd almost never be called to the coronary care unit to see people with diabetes. Of course, organisationally, lots of things have changed in the meantime. People with major heart attacks are taken not to their local general hospital, but to a cardiac centre for immediate treatment, so we don't see the people with diabetes who have the severest form of heart attacks. But even in our hospital diabetes clinics, I latterly saw fewer people who'd been discharged recently after a heart attack. I think there was also a decrease in the 'classical' symptom of angina – chest discomfort or shortness of breath on exertion developing over weeks or months. Angina usually indicates slowly progressing blockages of coronary arteries, rather than the sudden blockages that occur in a heart attack, so my experience was that both these indicators of severe disease of the coronary arteries supplying the heart muscle were becoming less common in people with diabetes.

But are my personal observations just wishful thinking? No, because they're borne out by the facts. For example, in the United States, the rate of heart attack (officially 'myocardial infarction' or 'MI' for short) in people with diabetes fell by one-half between 1990 and 2010. At the same time strokes, amputations of the leg and kidney failure also fell by approximately the same amount (see Figure 9.1). All four complications are related to arterial disease (see Chapter 11). Let's start with heart attacks.

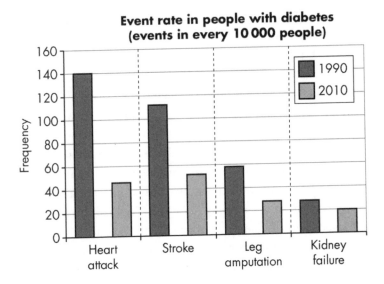

Figure 9.1: The dramatic reduction between 1990 and 2010 in the risk of serious vascular diseases in American people with Type 2 diabetes.

Heart attacks – a changing medical landscape in people with Type 2 diabetes

The observations in the USA and other countries that heart attack rates in diabetes have dramatically decreased over time don't tell us *why* these improvements have occurred, but it's probably because Type 2 people are looking after themselves better these days, and GPs in the UK are especially good at detecting and treating high blood pressure and cholesterol levels. So if the news is so great – is there still a problem? The major heart attacks that pole-axed my patients in the 1990s and brought them to the coronary care unit are less common now, but not all heart attacks are the classical ones associated with crushing pain in the centre of the chest, faintness, sweating, nausea and collapse, the typical symptoms of events caused by sudden blockage (occlusion) of a major artery to the heart. And it's the non-classical ones that are now more common, resulting in a dramatic change in the picture of heart disease in Type 2 diabetes.

The medical names given to these less dramatic heart attack events are complicated and keep changing. In fact even 'myocardial infarction' has been superseded by a broader term – 'acute coronary syndrome' (ACS). One particular type of myocardial infarction or ACS seems to particularly affect Type 2 patients – the so-called NSTEMI (most doctors can't remember what it stands for – 'non-ST segment elevation myocardial infarction' – so just remember it as an 'en-stemmy'). An NSTEMI can be associated with some chest discomfort, but equally there could be shortness of breath or generalised mild chest tightness (or, of course, the 'indigestion' that isn't indigestion). Often these minor symptoms go away of their own accord and at least in the short term nobody is any the wiser. A standard ECG heart tracing taken even shortly after the onset of these symptoms may not be dramatically abnormal, so we now use blood tests rather than the ECG to help decide whether there has been any damage to heart muscle, which is after all the important consequence of a heart attack. Using these tests we can now detect even minor heart damage that may not register on the ECG tracing, and it looks as if it is very common in Type 2. Minor heart damage means there is some underlying disease in the coronary arteries supplying the heart muscle – not so much blockages in the major arteries, but more likely minor blockages in the smaller arteries.

Key point: Major heart attacks are now less common, probably because self-care of diabetes has improved and we use medication effectively.

This picture of several areas of blockage in more than one of the three major coronary arteries is probably due to damage over a long period, perhaps decades (see Figure 9.2). A combination of abnormal cholesterol, blood pressure and glucose plus age (and smoking) all take a cumulative toll on the artery walls. When detailed tests are done of the heart structure in people with Type 2 diabetes, they seem to have had more overall damage, possibly through a greater number of these minor or undetected heart attacks, than people without diabetes.

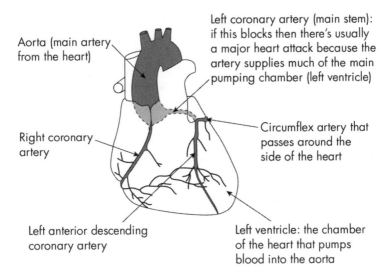

Figure 9.2: The main coronary arteries of the heart.

Smaller heart attacks and heart failure

Smaller heart attacks that people may not always be aware of cause progressive minor damage to the muscle of the heart. In the end, these recurrent small insults result in a heart that is less efficient at pumping out blood to the rest of the body. If the damage becomes too severe (for example, if less than about 45% of the main pumping chamber, the left ventricle, is working), then fluid tends to accumulate in the lungs, resulting in shortness of breath, and also in the legs, resulting in swelling of the ankles. This combination of symptoms is more common than before, especially in women and in ethnic minorities. Treatment of heart failure has hugely improved over the years and most hospital cardiology teams have appointed nurses who specialise in managing medication and lifestyle aspects of heart failure. Specialised exercise training can improve symptoms and cardiac function and sophisticated pacemakers are increasingly used to boost the function of the heart and improve breathing and tiredness.

> **Key point:** Minor heart attacks often go unrecognised but their cumulative effect can be to weaken the pumping muscle of the heart, leading to an increased risk of heart failure.

Heart attacks in ethnic minorities and women

Ethnic minorities

There has always been concern that ethnic minority people, especially from India, Pakistan and Bangladesh (south Asians), have a particularly high risk of heart attacks, whether or not they have diabetes. The reasons are complex and not fully understood, but there's little evidence that 'diet' is the problem, nor exercise, because when it is measured (see Chapter 8 References, page 225), Asian people are just as active (or inactive) as white Brits, and also when asked about how much exercise they take they are less likely to fib. As in white people, heart attacks in Type 2 south Asians have changed – but even more dramatically. A large UK study published in 2016 found that younger Asians who have heart disease have better outcomes and live longer than their white counterparts – and have a longer life expectancy. Older Asian people over 65 not only have less cardiovascular disease than their white counterparts, but there are also lower risks of cancer and of lung disease. Again, it's not easy to work out why these dramatic changes have occurred but it's likely to be due to a combination of increased individual and community awareness of the risk of heart disease, combined with better self-care and medical care. (Clarified butter – ghee – was previously blamed for the excess heart disease in south Asian people, and people are certainly eating less of it, but explanations are never as simple as that: most white British people studiously avoid butter these days, while the French eat at least three times as much butter as us and have very few heart attacks.)

There's less information on black people originating from Africa and the Caribbean, but heart attack rates are consistently much lower than in white UK people, though strokes are more common, probably because of their tendency to have high blood pressure.

Gender

The improvements in heart attack rates in Type 2 people have been less dramatic in women compared with men. There's a puzzle here that hasn't been fully solved. Non-diabetic women rarely have heart attacks (or strokes) before the menopause; once past the menopause they acquire the same risks as men of the same age. Even before they go through the menopause, Type 2 women have the same risk as younger men, and once past the menopause, they also have a high risk of the heart failure we just mentioned. In the past, after a heart attack, women were less likely to get an angiogram, coronary stent or bypass operation than men. Fortunately, this is no longer the case, but there continues to be concern that there is still less awareness of the *possibility* of coronary heart disease and the risk factors associated with it in women. If there are symptoms of heart disease – chest discomfort, shortness of breath or fatigue on exertion – then whatever your gender, it's equally likely to be heart trouble.

Technological interventions in the heart: stents and bypass surgery

Another huge change: when I was first a consultant, someone with diabetes who needed surgery to bypass blocked coronary arteries (coronary artery bypass graft, CABG, 'cabbage') often wouldn't get it, because it was thought to be too risky. All that's changed. One or two blocked arteries can usually be unblocked using a non-surgical procedure, where the coronary arteries are first X-rayed in detail by injecting a contrast liquid ('dye'). This is an 'angiogram'. The arteries can then be unblocked using a small balloon which is inflated in the blocked artery ('angioplasty'). Finally, a flexible tube (stent) is placed within the previously blocked segment. The stent keeps the artery open so that blood can flow freely through it. This is the 'angioplasty and stent' procedure. Nearly all stents are coated with a drug on their inner surface where they come into contact with blood in the coronary artery. The coating is one of a group of drugs that reduce inflammation and the tendency for blood to clot around the stent, and the drug is slowly released over many months. Stents have improved immeasurably over the past 20 years and so has the expertise of cardiologists to get them into the perfect position.

Do people with one or two coronary blockages always need stents? A couple of clinical trials, including the COURAGE study, have compared very intensive non-interventional management with the results of stent placement in people with one or two coronary blockages. Obsessive attention to exercise, diet, smoking cessation (of course), and keeping blood pressure, cholesterol and blood glucose under control is likely to be as good as stents at preventing future heart attacks (see References, page 226). This is an area where more evidence is genuinely needed, and a major study is due to report in 2019. But it again highlights the power of lifestyle changes to improve arterial disease.

Chapter 9

When do you need a bypass?

Now that stent placement is so much easier and has such good outcomes, if you had diabetes and three, four or more coronary blockages, what's to stop you having a trio or quartet of stents placed? The answer emerged gradually from several studies: if you have multiple arterial blockages, then although there was a very small risk of complications from a coronary bypass operation, the long-term benefits were greater than if you had lots of stents. It had been widely predicted that in the face of stent technology, heart surgeons would no longer be needed for bypass procedures. These studies ensured that heart surgeons, and in many cases their patients too, got a new spring in their step.

Bypass surgery used to be a major procedure involving a long hospital stay. That's changed and coronary bypass surgery is now straightforward, the progress fuelled by major improvements in anaesthetics, and what cardiac surgeons use to bypass the blocked coronary segments: previously veins taken from the leg, but where blood flow is especially important, small arteries near the breastbone are used.

Key point: The outlook for people who need stents or have a coronary bypass is improving all the time. If several coronary arteries are involved, bypass is especially beneficial in people with diabetes.

Lifestyle changes after a heart attack, stent or bypass

Cardiologists and heart surgeons are very competent at unblocking or bypassing arteries, but once they've done their high-tech bit, then it's over to equally important but less impressive technology to minimise the risk of further blockages and another heart attack. At this stage, everyone must become a permanent non-smoker. In addition, there's a portfolio of must-take medication, including a statin, aspirin and/or clopidogrel, a beta blocker and an ACE inhibitor (page 160). Just as important are dietary changes – for example, moving to the Mediterranean diet – but possibly the most important individual intervention is the cardiac rehabilitation programme.

The evidence for the benefits of cardiac rehabilitation is overwhelming. People who diligently complete the programme reduce the risk of another hospital admission by about 40%, and of a fatal heart attack by 25%. But cardiac rehabilitation is tough. In the COURAGE study, people were expected to do 30 to 45 minutes of moderate intensity exercise (for example, two miles of brisk walking) five times a week. In addition (see Chapter 8) all daily lifestyle activity must increase too – for example, taking the stairs rather than the escalator. After a formal rehabilitation course in Denmark, blood glucose and pressure levels both improved meaningfully and, not surprisingly, so did exercise capacity.

Identifying heart disease in diabetes

In spite of the major and highly welcome improvements in heart disease in Type 2s, it remains a problem. We've discussed above the fact that Type 2 people don't always get typical 'heart attack' symptoms or even classical angina when they over-exert themselves, but still may have coronary artery disease that risks damaging the heart. Can we identify people at risk of a heart attack before the event?

There's been a huge debate about this, and the short answer is: if you get no symptoms suggesting coronary trouble (in particular, chest discomfort on exertion and shortness of breath) there isn't a test that will detect if you have significant narrowing of the coronary arteries short of having a coronary angiogram, which is complicated, not without risk and certainly couldn't be done in large numbers of people. There have been several clinical trials, including the DIAD study. They recruited large groups of middle-aged Type 2 patients with nothing to suggest the presence of heart disease, and then divided them into a group that was tested with quite sophisticated scanning methods, and a group that was followed up without an initial test, but of course who would have them if they developed any symptoms. There was no overall difference in outcome – in either the number of people who died or who had heart attacks. Once again, the encouraging fact to emerge was that fewer than 1% of people developed any obvious heart symptoms during the follow-up, regardless of their allocated group. This shows – again – that Type 2 patients are looking after themselves very well these days, supported by their general practice teams.

Calculate your QRISK score of heart disease

The best way of predicting your risk is a scoring system developed in the UK – QRISK3 – visit https://qrisk.org/three/. To get the most accurate estimate, you need some measurements. Most people will know their height and weight (but height has to be in centimetres and weight in kilograms). In addition, you will need:

- Systolic blood pressure (see Chapter 10) – the upper number, so if your blood pressure is 134/76, enter 134.
- Total cholesterol and HDL cholesterol levels. These will be measured with your routine annual blood tests. Request the most recent measurements from your GP's records.

You'll know all the other requested information – but if you don't have it readily to hand, just leave the box blank.
You get two pieces of information:
- The first is your estimated risk of cardiovascular disease (this covers heart attack and stroke) over the next 10 years,

---

and is shown as a percentage. You'll also see a simple but clever graphic of smileys: yellow for people estimated not to have trouble in the next 10 years, interspersed with blue not-so-smileys representing people who are likely to run into trouble. I've just calculated mine and it's 13.5%, about one in 14, so that means slightly over 1% chance each year. A 10-year risk of 10% or higher is considered significant and worthy of extra-diligent preventive treatment.

- The second calculation puts your risk in context. In other words, are you more likely or less likely to have a heart attack than someone of your age who has no extra risk factors, and doesn't have Type 2? Again, I am slightly more likely to have an event compared with people of my age who have no risk factors at all (the ratio is 1.1, so overall a 10% increased risk).

(You may wonder why the questionnaire asks for your postcode. People in more deprived parts of the country have a higher risk of heart disease. The QRISK database uses your postcode as a rough indication of deprivation.)

Key point: Estimate your coronary/stroke risk with the QRISK calculator. The higher the risk the greater the benefit of exercise, weight loss, and excellent control of LDL cholesterol, blood pressure and blood glucose.

Other arterial troubles

Stroke

A colleague specialising in elderly care always called strokes 'brain attacks', a very good description, because like heart attacks, which result from a sudden blockage in one of the coronary arteries, a stroke is caused by a sudden blockage of one of the arteries supplying blood to the brain. The clever FAST campaign in the UK aimed to increase awareness of the early symptoms of stroke – it stands for Face weakness, Arm weakness, Slurred speech, Time (phone 999 quickly) – and raised awareness of how important it is to act FAST, because brain damage can often be reduced, and sometimes effectively stopped, if clot-busting drugs can be given within six hours of the onset of symptoms. More recently, fishing out the clot in the artery – just like they do in the case of a major heart attack – has proved to be valuable in reducing disability after a stroke, but it requires major resources to have the specialists on hand 24 hours a day to do these complicated procedures.

One of the difficulties of spotting stroke symptoms early on is that, like heart attacks, they are more likely to occur during the night, and although few people can remain asleep through an episode of crushing central chest discomfort, they may not be woken if they're having a stroke. This means that they wake up with a completed stroke, often outside the time-frame where clot-busting drugs are of value.

The risk of stroke is falling in non-diabetic and diabetic people (see Figure 9.1), and there are various reasons for this, many of them similar to the reasons for the reduction in heart attacks – for example, reduced levels of smoking, and better control of blood pressure and cholesterol levels. As we saw in Chapter 7, the reduction in strokes is also in part due to our eating less salt (though we still eat far too much). However, strokes are still a major cause of long-term disability, and because of the general increased risk of vascular disease in diabetes, they still occur about twice as frequently compared with non-diabetic people. The arterial disease which causes strokes is the same as in heart attacks, but different arteries become blocked – usually the large arteries of the neck (the carotid arteries), but, just as in heart attacks, more often now the smaller arteries in the brain itself.

We saw earlier that major heart attacks are much less common than 20 years ago, but there seems to have been no reduction in smaller events that may not be so obvious. The same goes for strokes. Smaller events are very common. These include mini-strokes (TIAs, or transient ischaemic attacks, where stroke-like symptoms resolve within a day), and small permanent strokes occurring just below the surface of the brain and in its deeper parts. By definition a TIA won't show up on a scan, but the smaller permanent events do, and a brain MRI scan will show them up as 'white spots'. As they accumulate over time, they may contribute to the increased risk of dementia/Alzheimer's-like conditions in Type 2s.

Preventing further events after an initial stroke is just as important as preventing further heart attacks, and the same interventions are required. But we don't so as well with stroke patients, where it's especially important to achieve systolic blood pressures of 130 mm or lower, keep total cholesterol levels to 3 mmol/l or lower, and LDL cholesterol to 2 or lower.

Key point: After a stroke, maintaining good glucose control (but without any hint of hypoglycaemia), blood pressure below 130 mm and cholesterol at 3 mmol/l or below is extremely important to reduce the risk of further events.

Looking after your blood pressure is the key to preventing strokes

As blood pressure goes up, the risk of heart attacks increases slightly, but the relationship between high blood pressure and stroke is much more powerful. Keeping blood pressure under control is the key to reducing the risk of a first stroke and reducing the risk of another stroke. Blood glucose control has very little impact on reducing stroke risk. We've seen that most people with Type 2 need blood pressure medication, but intensive attention to lifestyle is critically important as well (see Chapter 7). Until recently, many people with Type 2 took low-dose aspirin in the hope that it would reduce the risk of a first stroke, but any benefit is very small and the current view is that the risk of bleeding with aspirin is too high to warrant everyone with diabetes taking it. Of course, everyone who has had a definite stroke of any severity (including a TIA) benefits from daily low-dose aspirin (75 mg daily in the UK, 81 mg in the USA).

Key point: High blood pressure is the most important single risk factor for stroke. Systolic blood pressure in all people with diabetes should be lower than 140 mm, and possibly nearer 130.

Peripheral vascular disease affecting the legs and feet

Peripheral vascular disease results from blockages in the major arteries to the legs. They are huge arteries, supplying blood to the largest muscles in the body, and run all the way from the groin right down to the foot. Blockages can therefore occur at various different points. They are more prone to occurring where arteries branch off, so the key problem areas lie in the groin where the major artery (femoral) divides into two, and at the knee where the femoral artery divides into three vessels that supply the calf, ankle and foot. If the blockage in a large artery occurs suddenly there is terrible pain, and the leg becomes blue or pale. As in major heart attacks and strokes, this is much less commonly seen now, probably because more people than ever have given up smoking.

More gradual narrowing of the arteries, where some blood flow gets through, is still common. It causes cramps while walking (claudication), when the muscles of the leg need more blood than the narrowed arteries can supply. Narrowing of the arteries below

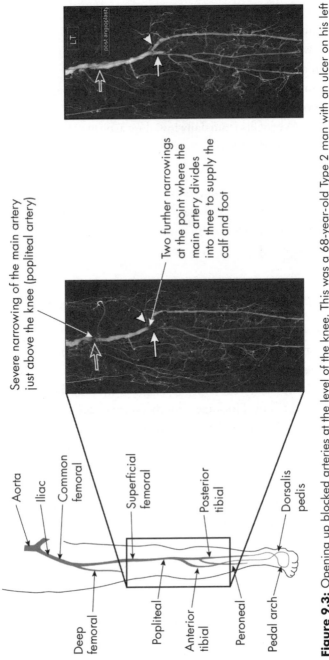

Figure 9.3: Opening up blocked arteries at the level of the knee. This was a 68-year-old Type 2 man with an ulcer on his left foot that wasn't healing because of insufficient blood supply. The left-hand diagram shows the arteries supplying blood to the foot. The X-ray picture in the middle shows the sites of three arterial blockages. On the right is the improved blood flow after the radiologist had opened up the blocked areas. The ulcer then healed within a few weeks. The X-rays were kindly supplied by Dr Sandeep Pathak and Dr Sergei Kuzmich, Whipps Cross University Hospital, London.

Severe narrowing of the main artery just above the knee (popliteal artery)

Two further narrowings at the point where the main artery divides into three to supply the calf and foot

Aorta

Iliac

Common femoral

Superficial femoral

Posterior tibial

Dorsalis pedis

Deep femoral

Popliteal

Anterior tibial

Peroneal

Pedal arch

the knee is especially common in Type 2 people, leading to cold feet, and sometimes to ulceration of the feet.

Like the coronary arteries, narrowed blood vessels to the legs can be opened up in one of two ways: angioplasty (and if necessary a stent to ensure the vessel remains open), or bypass. Radiologists – X-ray doctors – are the experts in angioplasty and stent placement (see Figure 9.3). Bypass surgery is much less used these days, but it still has a place in complicated cases.

Summary

Arterial disease causing heart attacks, strokes and pain and ulceration of the feet is now much less common in Type 2 diabetes than it was 20 years ago, but it is still the most important complication, and people with Type 2 remain at higher risk than non-diabetic people. Techniques of angioplasty, stents and bypass surgery have improved, but for the best outcomes with the lowest risk of further arterial troubles, secondary prevention with medication, diet, smoking cessation and exercise have been shown to reduce events by up to 50%. Smoking rates should be much lower in Type 2 than in the general population (currently about 16%) but we may not be achieving these.

Chapter 10

Blood pressure and cholesterol

Key points

Blood pressure

- High blood pressure (hypertension) affects the same organs as high blood glucose levels – so blood pressure needs just as much attention as blood glucose (but doesn't always get it).
- Systolic (upper) blood pressure in Type 2s should be between 130 and 140 mm Hg. The lower (diastolic) measurements are no longer considered relevant to long-term outcomes.
- Good self-care in blood pressure means taking your own measurements at home using reliable equipment.
- All blood pressure medication is safe, and has been in use for at least 20 years.
- Good blood pressure control meaningfully reduces the risk of strokes, heart attacks and worsening kidney function – and the benefit is greater in Type 2s than in people without diabetes.

Cholesterol

- The 'natural' total cholesterol level in groups who are at very low risk of heart attacks and strokes is about 3 mmol/l, compared with an average level of 5 in adults. The comparable values of LDL cholesterol – considered the most damaging fraction of cholesterol – are below 2 mmol/l.
- Diet and lifestyle can help a little, but very few people can reach the necessary low values without medication.
- Statins reduce the risk of vascular events by about 40% in people with diabetes.

- If possible, everyone who has had a heart attack or stroke should take a statin to get the LDL level to below 2 mmol/l.
- All other Type 2s should if possible also take a statin.
- Significant side-effects (especially involving the muscles) are very uncommon, but less serious side-effects are more common.
- Changing from one group of statins to another can help if you get side-effects.
- People who discontinue their statin on the basis of adverse reports in the press run a higher vascular risk. Discontinue only after a discussion with your medical team.

High blood pressure (hypertension)

Most people, even with very high blood pressure, will never experience any symptoms (everyone gets occasional headaches and dizziness), so, as with blood glucose and cholesterol, numbers are critical. Agreeing on those numbers – much like glucose and cholesterol – is another matter, but over the past few years, a general consensus has developed that people with diabetes should always have blood pressure measurements lower than 140/80 mm Hg and people who already have some complications, especially kidney, should have measurements that are nearer 130/80 mm. The 'mm Hg' refers to the old method of measuring blood pressure with a mercury-filled gauge, so 'mm' means millimetres of mercury (Hg). (Officially blood pressure numbers should be recorded as 'mm Hg' – Hg being the chemical symbol for mercury; but I have generally restricted it to 'mm' throughout the book.)

Doctors don't help Type 2 people by often making the numbers more complicated than they need be. We still record two blood pressure numbers separated by a slash, for example 145/80. Up to about 20 years ago the number after the slash – the 'diastolic' value – was thought to be the most important one in determining the risk of the serious outcomes of high blood pressure, heart attacks, strokes and kidney disease (see Figure 10.1). Clinical trials of blood pressure control in the early 1990s still focused on achieving low diastolic measurements, while the first, higher number (the 'systolic' pressure) was mostly ignored. This has completely changed now, and every recent clinical trial has used only the systolic measurement. But doctors are terrible creatures of habit; while diastolic pressure measurements are almost irrelevant, we still always measure it, and even clinical trials that focus only on systolic blood pressure targets still measure and quote the diastolics. There are silly 'rules' as well, still occasionally quoted by doctors – for example, the idea that your systolic blood pressure should be lower than your age plus 100. Silly – and dangerous. For example, no person aged 60, diabetic or not, should have a systolic blood pressure of 160. Actually, it's probably too high for a 90-year-old. Ditch this myth as well as all the others. Blood pressure is now really simple.

> **Key point:** Systolic blood pressure should always be lower than 140 mm. Aim for around 130 if you've had a stroke or heart attack or if your kidneys have been stressed by diabetes. Ignore the lower diastolic number.

Measure your own blood pressure

For the remainder of this section I'm going to be radical and stop even mentioning diastolic blood pressure: from now on, I'll only mention systolic pressures. Remember, they should always be under 140 mm.

In Type 2s not taking insulin there is still an unresolved discussion about the value of finger-prick blood glucose monitoring. The discussion will continue until we do a large clinical trial, and the wait may be a long one. Fortunately, when it comes to home-monitoring of blood pressure, the trials have been done and the answers are clear: it's not only easy to measure your own blood pressure, but the measurements are highly reliable, and – most important of all – they're more meaningful than those taken, often in haste, in the stressed environment of a hospital or general

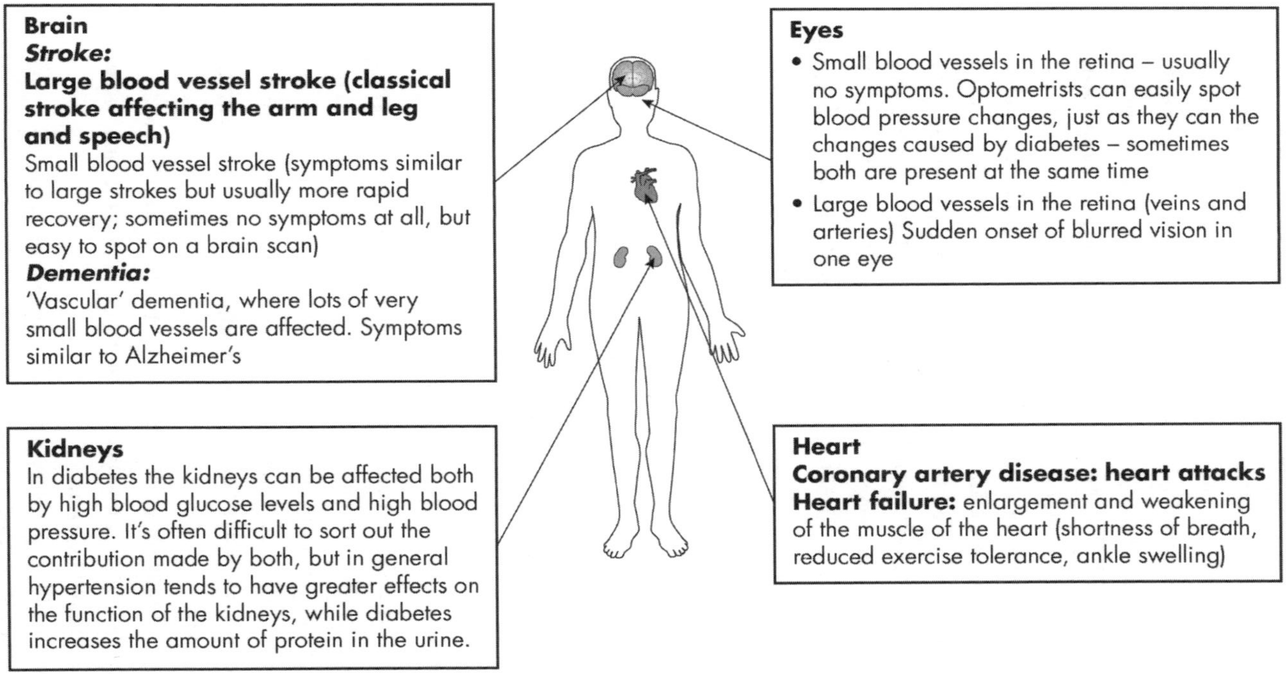

Figure 10.1: The effects of high blood pressure. These are broadly the same whether or not you have diabetes, but in Type 2 the risk of these complications is higher.

Eyes
- Small blood vessels in the retina – usually no symptoms. Optometrists can easily spot blood pressure changes, just as they can the changes caused by diabetes – sometimes both are present at the same time
- Large blood vessels in the retina (veins and arteries) Sudden onset of blurred vision in one eye

Heart
Coronary artery disease: heart attacks
Heart failure: enlargement and weakening of the muscle of the heart (shortness of breath, reduced exercise tolerance, ankle swelling)

Brain
Stroke:
Large blood vessel stroke (classical stroke affecting the arm and leg and speech)
Small blood vessel stroke (symptoms similar to large strokes but usually more rapid recovery; sometimes no symptoms at all, but easy to spot on a brain scan)
Dementia:
'Vascular' dementia, where lots of very small blood vessels are affected. Symptoms similar to Alzheimer's

Kidneys
In diabetes the kidneys can be affected both by high blood glucose levels and high blood pressure. It's often difficult to sort out the contribution made by both, but in general hypertension tends to have greater effects on the function of the kidneys, while diabetes increases the amount of protein in the urine.

practice clinic, giving rise to 'white coat hypertension' or 'the white coat effect'. Clinic measurements are usually significantly higher than home measurements, perhaps by as much as 10 mm.

You just need the right equipment, and to take the minimum number of measurements in the correct way. The equipment is easy to deal with. For people in the UK, the British Hypertension Society keeps an updated list of validated equipment on its website (see References, page 228). It strongly recommends equipment that uses an arm cuff; devices with wrist or finger cuffs are not approved because blood pressure measurements are reliable only if they are taken at the level of the heart. Omron, Boots and Lloyds devices are the most familiar in the UK. They are usually on offer at £20 or less. Equipment that stores readings electronically is more expensive, and it's best to get the simplest device and write down your blood pressure readings (or store them on your phone).

> **Key point:** Home blood pressure equipment should have arm cuffs – not wrist (or even finger) cuffs, which don't measure blood pressure reliably.

How and when to take your own blood pressure

There are lots of different recommendations. Blood pressure is highest first thing in the morning, and then settles, so take measurements later in the day – for example, late morning and evening.

- Take two measurements at about the same time of day for five to seven days before a clinic appointment or meeting your GP.
- Do a similar series of measurements about four weeks after starting a new medication or changing the dose of an existing medication.
- If your blood pressure and medication are stable, a measurement series every six months is fine.

- Don't measure your blood pressure if you're stressed or in pain, and before taking it sit quietly and comfortably in a chair with your feet flat on the ground (crossing your legs often increases blood pressure).
- Make sure your upper arm is bare – no tight sleeves.
- Use the same arm for each measurement. The right is usually used, but attaching the cuff requires some skill, so the left arm is fine for right-handed people. Make sure the cuff covers the bend in the elbow and that the arrow on the cuff is situated over the inner side of the elbow – nearest the body.
- Take two measurements a minute apart.
- Write down the measurements.

Key point: If you're taking medication for high blood pressure, aim to do your blood pressure regularly – though not necessarily frequently – at home.

'Low' blood pressure

All doctors in diabetes clinics have heard from slightly panicked patients that they were told their blood pressure was found to be 'low'. Is that a good or bad thing? The answer is … it depends.

I apologise for this entirely predictable 'medical' response, but please don't chuck the book away in irritation; it took a long time to write. The 'low' blood pressure story has had a few twists and turns. First, let's consider what is 'normal' blood pressure in a younger person who's not taking blood pressure medication. Simple: it's 120 mm or lower (120/80 or lower if you insist). There are countless young (usually slim) people, entirely fit and well who have even lower pressures – for example 90 or 100 mm. They're in robust good health, and are likely to live to a ripe old age; their whole circulation is gentle and low pressure, but working very well, and their blood vessels won't be stressed.

However, most of us aren't in either of these categories: we're no longer young, and we're taking blood pressure medication, and that's where 'low' blood pressure might not be such a good thing. In several clinical trials, Type 2s taking medication, often older people in their 60s, and who have pressures of 120 mm or lower, have a slightly *increased* risk of heart attacks and other vascular events, and once the pressures fall to 110 or lower, then the kidneys can be stressed as well. In addition, these low pressures can give unpleasant symptoms – for example, dizziness, especially when standing up or getting out of bed in the morning. So: aim for a blood pressure under 140 mm, but avoid 120 or lower.

> **Key point:** The target systolic blood pressure in people with diabetes is ideally between 120 and 140 mm. It shouldn't go below 110 mm.

Treatment of hypertension

Drug treatment

We've seen that hypertension is hazardous and more so in Type 2s than in non-diabetic people. Non-drug approaches to hypertension were discussed in Chapter 7. Drug treatment of high blood pressure is effective and works very quickly. It reduces the risk of stroke and heart attack, and in the longer term helps preserve kidney function. For reasons that are still not clear, but possibly related to insulin resistance and the metabolic syndrome (see Chapter 3), Type 2 diabetes and hypertension go hand in hand, so that before treatment about 80% of Type 2s have systolic blood pressure above 140 mm. It's a very unusual Type 2 hypertensive individual who can get away with no blood pressure medication at all, and many need two, three, four or even more medications. If there are kidney problems, especially protein in the urine (see Chapter 11), medication is critical for preserving good kidney function. Specific non-drug interventions, especially the DASH diet, and reducing salt and alcohol intake, can help you reduce the number or doses of blood pressure tablets you need (see Chapter 7), but don't expect to be able to ditch every blood pressure medication; by the time most of us develop Type 2 diabetes in our late 50s or early 60s, hypertension has often been present for as long as 30 years.

As we discussed in Chapter 7, medication for blood pressure doesn't cause as much anxiety as blood sugar medication or drugs for cholesterol (see the statin story below), and this is largely because drugs used for hypertension are old and well established. There have been a few attempts to introduce new drugs in the past 15–20 years, but they were either withdrawn or stopped being used because of side-effects right from the start, and it's unlikely we'll see many more. But there's a lot more we can do with existing (and sometimes very old and relatively unused) drugs, especially if used in logical combinations. This is particularly important in about 10% of Type 2s (amounting to a large total number of patients) whose blood pressure is difficult to control. We'll briefly look at this phenomenon – 'resistant' hypertension – below. Table 10.1 lists the main categories of blood pressure medication.

Table 10.1: Major groups of blood pressure medication

Type of medication	Examples of widely used drugs (generic – chemical – names)	Comments
ACE inhibitors (ACE = angiotensin converting enzyme)	Ramipril, lisinopril, perindopril	Highly protective for kidneys in people with Type 2 diabetes and protein in the urine. Introduced in the 1970s and '80s; some of the most important drugs in modern use. Particular side effect: cough.
ARB (angiotensin receptor blockers)	Losartan, irbesartan, candesartan	Similar to the ACE inhibitors and also protective in people with diabetic kidney disease. Introduced in the 1980s and 1990s. Cough isn't a side-effect, but both ACE inhibitors and ARB drugs can cause allergies. They raise the level of potassium in the blood, so occasional blood tests are needed.
Calcium channel blockers	Amlodipine, lercanidipine, diltiazem	Very effective drugs, introduced in the 1970s and '80s. If Type 2s require two different medications for blood pressure, then an ACE inhibitor (or ARB), together with a calcium channel blocker is by far the most common combination. Few side-effects: headaches when you start taking them, swollen ankles and very occasionally swollen gums occur at high doses.

Diuretics	Indapamide, bendroflumethiazide	The first antihypertensive drugs to be introduced from the 1950s onwards. Very effective drugs, especially in combination with other classes. Nearly always the third drug in a triple combination.
	'Potassium-sparing' diuretics e.g. spironolactone, amiloride	Very valuable in combination with another diuretic in people with 'resistant' hypertension.
Beta blockers	Atenolol, bisoprolol, metoprolol, carvedilol, nebivolol	Extremely versatile drugs, discovered in the UK in the 1970s. Beneficial in people who have had heart attacks and angina. Very important in heart failure. Less used now in hypertension because of well-known side-effects (e.g. tiredness, cold hands and feet, erectile dysfunction).
Doxazosin (alpha blocker)	Doxazosin is the only one currently used	Effective in people intolerant of other drugs. The most recent drug to be introduced – but still 20 years old. The slow-release (modified-release) form is the most effective.

The drudgery of taking blood pressure medication

Although taking two, three or more medications for anything is a chore, it may be some consolation to know that not very many years ago, blood pressure medication had to be taken twice or even three times a day. All antihypertensive medication is now once-daily. Blood pressure tends to be higher first thing in the morning, so taking your medication late at night or at bedtime may help, but morning medication is far better than forgetting to take it at night.

As with any drug treatment, some people discontinue medication; about one in five stop taking their tablets, for a variety of reasons (this seems to be particularly the case for the ACE inhibitor and ARB drugs compared with other types of medication, an unexpected finding as these groups have very few side-effects). Careful reviews with pharmacists can help increase regular tablet-taking.

People with hypertension often tell me they don't have time to take their tablets, and always reassure me that once they retire they'll have more time to look after themselves, and that would – of course – include absolutely regular medication-taking. Not so. A large study of people working in the Finnish public sector discovered that men and women alike were about one-third less likely to take their blood pressure medication after they retired (in men, though not women, this extended to not taking their diabetes medication either). Does this matter? Yes: in another study people admitted to hospital with a heart attack or stroke were more likely to die if they had previously taken less than 50% of their tablets (see References, page 228).

> **Key point:** Blood pressure rises even if you miss just one day's medication. Retired people may not be as good at taking their tablets as people in work.

Hypertension that's difficult to control

Resistant hypertension – hypertension that is difficult to control – is defined as blood pressure of 140 mm or higher in someone taking at least three medications, one of which must be a diuretic (diuretics help all other drugs to work better, especially if they're accompanied by a low-salt diet). It's a useful definition, because it alerts patients and doctors alike to the need for a careful medical assessment and medication review if blood pressure seems not to be well controlled. Some people turn out to have abnormal-looking adrenal glands (tiny organs perched on top of the kidneys), which can be overproducing a salt-retaining hormone called aldosterone. Blood tests, and perhaps also a CT scan of the adrenal glands, can identify an adrenal problem. But in most cases of resistant hypertension, a group of old drugs, actually diuretics themselves, has found a new lease of life, often with dramatic effects in reducing blood pressure (see Table 10.1). Their effect is greatly enhanced by intensive lifestyle measures, focusing on reducing salt intake (see Chapter 7).

Cholesterol

The cholesterol story has been running now for 70 years or more, and shows no sign of coming to an end – and certainly not a tidy end. Although there are still controversies over blood glucose and its links to the complications of Type 2, we have seen there are no street fights or headlines about blood pressure control. Why, then, has the war over cholesterol not come to a peaceful end? I think there are several reasons, all related to our poor understanding of the links between blood cholesterol, fats in food and heart attack risks. First, research, even after all this time, can't explain why there is only a weak link between blood cholesterol levels encountered in most of the population and vascular diseases (especially heart attack and stroke), but why *reducing* cholesterol levels with statins has such a dramatic effect on *reducing* that risk.

A second unresolved problem is the relationship between the saturated fat content of food, particularly animal products, and blood cholesterol levels. Food itself contains almost no cholesterol; plants can't manufacture cholesterol, so no vegetable contains any cholesterol. Eggs and other animal products contain small amounts, but much less than the quantities produced by the ever-versatile liver. Because food contains almost no cholesterol, it can't be responsible for high blood cholesterol. What does, then, cause high blood cholesterol levels? Much of it is genetic, and there's nothing we're going to be able to do about that for a very long time. The amount of saturated fats (quite different from cholesterol) in foods derived from animals has only a weak link with blood cholesterol level, and eaten in usual quantities, meat, for example, has only a small effect on blood cholesterol values.

The final weak link in this very feeble chain is that even if you make a huge dietary effort, or lose an enormous amount of weight, there isn't likely to be a major change in your blood cholesterol (see Chapter 7). For example, huge weight loss after bariatric surgery results in only a small reduction in total cholesterol levels. The level of harmful LDL cholesterol barely changes, and in some studies goes up. In the Look AHEAD study, in which Type 2 patients lost around 9 kg in the first year, and remained with 4–5 kg weight loss for at least four years, there were no changes in any of the cholesterol measurements.

Scientifically, all this uncertainty generates frustration and controversy, but only because we expect to be able to uncover simple links in medicine: too much 'sugar' in the diet 'causes' Type 2 diabetes (you now know that isn't the case); too much dietary 'fat' causes heart disease (but not if you're French). And so on. Nothing is that simple, so the best thing we can all do is wait for clinical science to try and sort out the whole confusing story, retain our wonder at the complexity of the way we function, and recognise the validity of highly important clinical outcome studies, such as PREDIMED, which confirmed the beneficial effect of the Mediterranean diet on something that is really important to Type 2s: reducing vascular damage. And although the Mediterranean diet is quite low in saturated fat – itself resulting in perhaps a small *reduction* in harm – the *benefits* of a high intake of polyunsaturated fats in the same diet are much greater.

Key point: We still don't fully understand the links between dietary fat, blood cholesterol levels and the risk of heart disease.

Fatty stuff other than cholesterol

Apart from cholesterol, there is a myriad of other fatty substances, lumped together as 'lipids', that circulate in the blood and interact with critical organs. Recall that carbohydrates generate fats called triglycerides, which get stored wherever they can be deposited, usually in the liver, but also in the pancreas, in muscle and other organs (see Chapters 1 and 3). Other lipids, including cholesterol itself, are used to manufacture cell walls, and are therefore needed in large amounts, as we are constantly regenerating new cells. There are hundreds of these complex long-chain chemicals, all interacting with one another and being modified from one to another. But in routine practice, we measure only a few of them:

- **Total cholesterol:** This is the number we're most likely to remember, though because it represents a mixture of different cholesterols it's not the best one for estimating cardiac risk. The 'normal' level used to be quoted as 5 mmol/l but that's the *average* level in a Western population, where heart disease is common. Laboratories have stopped quoting these arbitrary numbers, and as we'll see below, most people with Type 2 diabetes should be aiming for levels of 3 mmol/l or lower. The accolade for the number that reflects cardiac risk most directly belongs to LDL cholesterol.
- **LDL (low-density lipoprotein) cholesterol:** LDL cholesterol is only one component of total cholesterol and is about 60% lower than normal. LDL cholesterol level broadly correlates with the risk of coronary heart disease and other vascular diseases – the lower the number the lower the risk – and is the measurement (see below) that has become

the target for treatment in Type 2s. Just as 'normal' total cholesterol used to be quoted as 5 mmol/l, 'normal' LDL cholesterol was thought to be around 3 mmol/l. But we don't need guesswork to establish the kind of LDL levels we should be aiming for. There are good studies of real-life LDL levels in humans and animals who never get coronary heart disease. Whether you measure it in newborn babies, primates in the wild, other wild mammals and – perhaps most relevant of all – hunter-gatherer humans, the average LDL in all these groups is about 1.6 mmol/l (equivalent to a total cholesterol of about 3 mmol/l). In Western societies only a tiny number of adults have an LDL of 3, but clearly that's what we should be aiming for to lower the risk of heart attacks and strokes (see Figure 10.2).

- **HDL (high density lipoprotein) cholesterol:** As total cholesterol and LDL cholesterol levels rise, the risk of vascular complications broadly increases. But not all high levels of fats are 'bad'; the higher the HDL cholesterol level, the *lower* the risk, and this is because one of the functions of HDL cholesterol is to transport cholesterol around the body and store it out of harm's way. (Interestingly, people with Type 1 diabetes often have very high HDL levels, and those with the very highest levels tend to be protected against long-term complications.) Unfortunately Type 2s often have low HDL levels, and this is a more consistent finding than a higher total or LDL cholesterol (and is so characteristic of Type 2 and of pre-diabetes that a low HDL cholesterol is considered part of the metabolic syndrome – see Chapter 3). Like total and LDL cholesterol, diet seems to play a limited part in determining your individual HDL level, and genetics is probably the most important factor, though moderate alcohol intake and intensive exercise can increase HDL. Up to the time of the menopause, non-diabetic women have

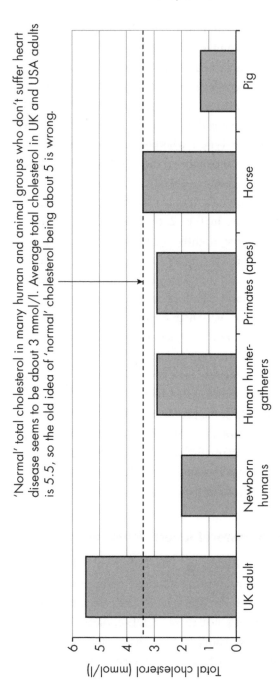

'Normal' total cholesterol in many human and animal groups who don't suffer heart disease seems to be about 3 mmol/l. Average total cholesterol in UK and USA adults is 5.5, so the old idea of 'normal' cholesterol being about 5 is wrong.

Figure 10.2: Total cholesterol levels in groups that have almost zero risk of heart attacks or strokes. You want to be more like them? Aim for a total cholesterol of 3 or lower.

higher HDL levels than men, and this goes a long way to explaining why younger non-diabetic women have a much lower risk of heart disease than their male counterparts. Type 2 diabetes erodes this differential, so that Type 2 men and women at all ages tend to have the same, lower, HDL levels. The message is that we need to look after the hearts of all people with Type 2 whether male or female.

• **Triglycerides:** We encountered these diet-derived fats early on in this book. They are only a very weak predictor of heart risk, and are only very occasionally high enough to pose a cardiac risk. In Type 2, they are only moderately raised (for example, slightly higher than 1.7 mmol/l, which is considered the upper limit of 'normal'), and this is probably more an indicator of nutritional overload and of pre-diabetes (and therefore of fatty liver) than an actual cardiac risk factor. Very high triglyceride levels (for example above 4 mmol/l) are sometimes seen in people who drink large amounts of alcohol, and there is a group of genetic disorders that can cause high levels, which in my experience in East London occurs quite often in young men of south Asian heritage. In some people, very high triglyceride levels, for unknown reasons, can attack the pancreas, resulting in painful and potentially hazardous pancreatitis, and eventually diabetes (because of the destruction of insulin-producing beta-cells in the islets).

Getting the cholesterol levels down: why bother?

The facts are simple. Reducing LDL cholesterol is more beneficial in the long term in preventing vascular diabetes complications than reducing blood glucose levels – and even than reducing blood pressure. That's not to say LDL cholesterol is the *only* game in town, but we should always have our beady eyes on it.

Intensive diet (see Chapter 7) focusing on nutraceuticals

known to reduce cholesterol levels may help a little. Reducing food intake in the Newcastle way will reduce triglycerides and reduce the risk of pre-diabetes and of fatty liver. But in most people these measures need support from medication – statins – in order to reduce the devastating vascular complications of Type 2, and that's where a very long media war of attrition has been going on. But before joining the battle, let's take a look at the evidence. First, we've just seen that animals and people who are at zero risk of heart disease naturally have very low levels of cholesterol and LDL. Do similar levels of cholesterol and LDL offer protection in people with Type 2?

The CARDS study (2004)

The CARDS study changed the way we thought about statin treatment in Type 2. Several studies way back in the late 1980s had already shown quite clearly that statin treatment in people who'd already had a heart attack reduced their risk of dying from another heart attack. So there was no controversy that statin treatment after a heart attack was life-saving. The medical term for treatment of this group of people who'd already had a hospital admission with a heart attack or stroke is *secondary* prevention – how can we prevent a second (and subsequent) event?

But the remaining question, which would apply to a much larger group of people, was whether reducing cholesterol levels in people who had not yet had a heart attack or stroke (*primary* prevention) could reduce the risk of either event happening in the first place. CARDS was therefore a simple study. It used the statin called atorvastatin in a low dose (10 mg daily): half the patients took the statin daily for four years while the remainder took the placebo dummy drug.

These are the blood lipid levels in the CARDS study (all values in mmol/l).

	Total cholesterol	LDL cholesterol
Value at the start of the trial	5.4	3.0
At end of the trial (taking statin)	4.0	1.8
Reduction	-1.4	-1.2

At the start you can see the average cholesterol was not especially high – just over 5 mmol/l. Within a few months of the start of the trial, Type 2s taking atorvastatin were already having fewer vascular events (strokes and heart attacks) than those taking the placebo, but the trial had to continue until the statistics were convincing. After four years the combined risk of vascular events was reduced by 40% (see References, page 229). This was an even better result than anticipated, and from the mid-2000s nearly all Type 2s were encouraged to start long-term treatment with a statin. At the same time, the very high-risk people who'd had a heart attack or stroke were being encouraged, also on the basis of very strong evidence, that their risks would be lowered if they achieved levels similar to the ones we've seen in extremely low-risk groups – children and adults of native groups.

Key point: Statin treatment reduces the risks of heart attacks and strokes by nearly one-half in all people with Type 2 diabetes.

Statins, side-effects and the media battle

The only reliably effective way of getting total cholesterol levels down to 3 mmol/l and LDL to less than 2 is by regularly taking a statin. Other medications have been used, but even if they get the numbers down, they don't do what's really important – reduce vascular risk. Statins, like every other drug, have side-effects, but in addition to their genuine medical side-effects, the media have added to the concern about taking them. There is some evidence that when the media get into one of their periodic states over statins, they can influence people's medication taking.

To demonstrate what effect scare stories can have, the Danes did a very clever study. Danish people, like us in the UK, are concerned about the hazards and side-effects of statins. Researchers identified negative media stories about statins, and then from their extensive national health records identified people taking statins at the time, and followed up these people to see whether they discontinued their statins – and studied any possible medical consequences.

Scarily, but not too surprisingly, heart attack rates increased by about 25%, and cardiovascular death rates by about 18% in those who had discontinued their statin. The clear message is that stopping statin treatment is a medical decision to be taken between you and your medical team, and not one that should be in the hands of a newspaper (see References, page 227). We don't know enough individual detail about the reasons for the Danish people discontinuing statins, but it's much more likely to be the story than actual side-effects.

However, doctors and researchers haven't faced the problem of statin side-effects very well. They're old drugs now, and some were introduced in the 1980s when monitoring of side-effects during and after clinical trials wasn't as rigorous as it is now. The serious side-effects, mostly involving the muscles, became apparent very quickly, especially a very rare effect (almost literally one in a million) in which the muscles started breaking down and resulted in the kidneys shutting down. In my 35 years in the NHS I was aware of only one patient who had this serious side-effect, and he got through it without any lasting problems. Less serious muscle aches and pains are much more common, and if they are related to the statin they usually start in the first four weeks of treatment. Conversely, if they are related to the statin – we have many reasons for muscle aches and pains – then they will disappear within about two weeks of discontinuing.

The real problem isn't the severe side-effects which are always highlighted and feared. It's the less obvious symptoms that concern people because they continue with treatment, and since statins are lifelong treatment, even minor symptoms that go on for a long time could be cumulatively very troublesome. Because there will be no further clinical trials of statins we still don't really know the full spectrum of mild side-effects. They include 'flu-like symptoms, stomach problems and vivid dreams; but everyone gets these from time to time, so it's very difficult to sort out which ones are statin-related. Some people describe mild muddling of the brain (though statins definitely don't increase the risk of Alzheimer's – that's been investigated in detail, and in some studies there is a lower risk of memory problems in later life in people who take statins). There's no increased cancer risk: that's been followed up in huge numbers of patients. But there are several non-statin drugs that may increase the risk of side-effects when taken with a statin (some blood pressure medication, for example, including the calcium channel blockers). The interaction between statins and grapefruit and grapefruit juice is well known, but occasional grapefruit is unlikely to be a problem.

Four statins are used in the UK. Simvastatin is the one that is prescribed most often, because it was used in the early major clinical trials. Atorvastatin is similar to simvastatin, but more powerful in its cholesterol-reducing effects, and many people are now started on it, rather than simvastatin, especially as its patent expired several years ago, and therefore became much less expensive. Two less widely used drugs include pravastatin (relatively weak) and rosuvastatin (powerful). They are chemically different from simvastatin and atorvastatin, metabolised in a different way and seem to be less likely to give side-effects. If you've developed side-effects with simvastatin or atorvastatin, it's worthwhile changing to one of the other two.

> **Key point:** Although all medications properly used in Type 2 diabetes help reduce long-term complications, statins are the most effective.

Other cholesterol-lowering drugs

Ezetimibe

Apart from the newly-introduced PCSK9 inhibitors (see below), ezetimibe is the only non-statin drug that both reduces LDL levels and also the risk of vascular events, but it took many years for its cardiovascular benefits to be shown in a clinical trial. It's a fascinating drug, completely unrelated to the statins, and therefore with no statin side-effects. It works by reducing the amount of cholesterol absorbed from the gut, and is therefore similar to plant stanols/sterols in spreads and drinks (see Chapter 6). You may well ask: if there's not very much cholesterol in most of the foods we eat, how can it have such a powerful effect? The answer is that most of the cholesterol that ends up in the gut doesn't come from food, but is manufactured in the liver, where it passes as bile into the gall bladder which then empties into the gut. Ezetimibe works by preventing much of this own-manufacture cholesterol being absorbed. It's less powerful than statins, reducing LDL by about 15% (compared with up to 50% reduction with statins), but in the IMPROVE-IT trial reduced heart attack and stroke rates by the amount you'd expect with this degree of cholesterol-lowering. It's valuable in people who find it difficult to tolerate statins, and because it acts differently, it works very well in combination.

PCSK9 inhibitors

This is the most recent drug group, again completely different from statins. These drugs (examples include alirocumab and evolocumab) have to be taken by injection, much like insulin, but only every two or four weeks. (If you find these drug names impossible to pronounce, you're no different from most doctors.) They are as effective in lowering LDL cholesterol levels as the most powerful statins at their highest doses. They are also extremely expensive, and will for the foreseeable future be restricted to people with genetically very high levels of cholesterol and a very high risk of heart disease who are unable to tolerate any statin treatment. Do they reduce the risk of heart attacks and strokes? Probably. Are they safe? Again, probably. But we'll have to wait a good while for the 'excitement' that often surrounds these dramatic drugs to settle with the help of very large clinical trials, which are currently reporting.

Summary

In order to reduce the risk of vascular disease, all Type 2s need to aim for a systolic blood pressure between 130 and 140 mm, and an LDL cholesterol level under 2 mmol/l, corresponding to a total cholesterol lower than 3. Antihypertensive medication definitely reduces the risk of heart disease and stroke, so long as it's taken regularly. For lowering cholesterol some nutraceuticals may help a little, but nearly all Type 2s need long-term statin treatment to achieve adequate cholesterol levels that will reduce the risk of vascular events, especially stroke and heart attack. Careful choice of the right statin in most cases will avoid side-effects.

Chapter 11

Avoiding eye, kidney and nerve complications

Key points

- The most feared complications of diabetes are visual loss, kidney failure and amputation, due to Type 2 damaging small blood vessels in the eyes, kidney and nerves supplying the feet.
- The risk factors for these complications – high blood glucose, high blood pressure and high cholesterol – are the same as for heart attacks and strokes discussed in Chapter 9.
- Annual retinal photographs reliably identify early complications at the back of the eye – diabetic retinopathy. Severe eye complications have fallen since the national photographic screening programme was established in 2008.
- Annual blood and urine tests pick up early kidney complications (diabetic nephropathy), though they may not have been as successful in reducing serious complications as the eye programme. Fortunately, the risks of severe kidney disease have fallen over the past 20–30 years.
- Use the portfolio approach to prevent complications. Simple specific medication (for example, ACE inhibitors) combined with attention to blood glucose and cholesterol levels reduces the kidney risk, and probably helps the eyes too. Specialist eye doctors (ophthalmologists) now have sophisticated drugs, laser and advanced surgical techniques for the small number of people who develop serious retinopathy.
- We don't have specific treatments for most of symptoms caused by impaired nerve function in the legs (neuropathy), but looking after your feet very carefully does a lot to prevent serious complications.

Small vessel complications of diabetes

The impact of diabetes is mostly on blood vessels, and since blood vessels are everywhere, diabetes can have effects almost anywhere in the body. We discussed diabetes and the large artery complications – heart attacks, strokes and peripheral vascular disease affecting blood vessels to the legs and feet – in Chapter 9, but smaller blood vessels that supply the deeper parts of body structures are also affected. In most people, damage is minor or doesn't occur at all and has no long-term consequences, but some people develop progressive complications in the vessels of the retina of the eyes, or the kidneys, or the nerves, and vision and kidney function can be affected. Figure 11.1 summarises these complications, known collectively as 'microvascular' problems, that is, affecting small vessels.

Eyes (diabetic retinopathy)

The NHS has a good screening service for the specific retinal complications of diabetes, and in the UK and other countries where similar annual screening services have been established, the numbers of people losing vision from retinopathy have fallen dramatically. Even the most difficult retinal complication – maculopathy, which impairs vision because it involves the small area of the retina which we instinctively use to focus on fine details – is likely to become less common because there are new and highly specific drugs that, when given by injection directly into the eye, help stabilise the structure of the retina.

In gloomsville articles on complications written by 'experts', we always used to kick off with the shock-horror line: 'diabetic eye disease is the commonest cause of visual loss in people of working age'. Well, it isn't any longer, and in fact hasn't been since 2010. Although understandably feared, visual loss from diabetes is extremely rare these days. And that's been a massive change: when I first became a consultant in the mid-1990s, the

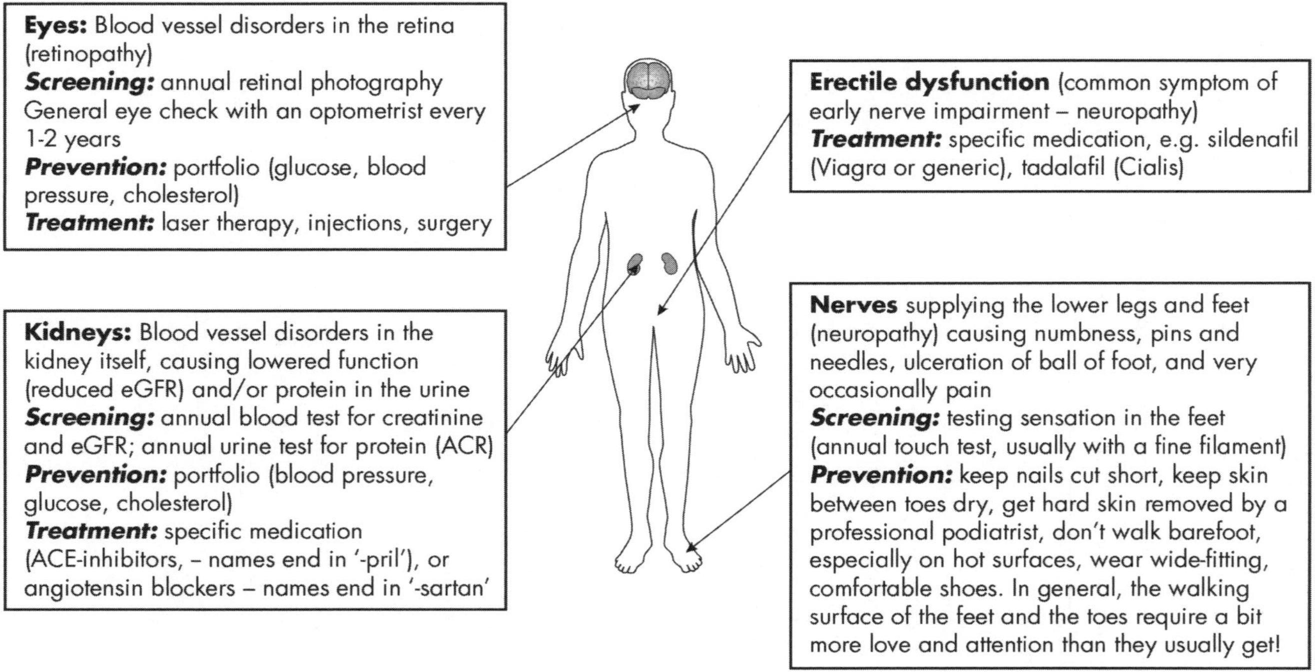

Eyes: Blood vessel disorders in the retina (retinopathy)
Screening: annual retinal photography General eye check with an optometrist every 1-2 years
Prevention: portfolio (glucose, blood pressure, cholesterol)
Treatment: laser therapy, injections, surgery

Kidneys: Blood vessel disorders in the kidney itself, causing lowered function (reduced eGFR) and/or protein in the urine
Screening: annual blood test for creatinine and eGFR; annual urine test for protein (ACR)
Prevention: portfolio (blood pressure, glucose, cholesterol)
Treatment: specific medication (ACE-inhibitors, – names end in '-pril'), or angiotensin blockers – names end in '-sartan'

Erectile dysfunction (common symptom of early nerve impairment – neuropathy)
Treatment: specific medication, e.g. sildenafil (Viagra or generic), tadalafil (Cialis)

Nerves supplying the lower legs and feet (neuropathy) causing numbness, pins and needles, ulceration of ball of foot, and very occasionally pain
Screening: testing sensation in the feet (annual touch test, usually with a fine filament)
Prevention: keep nails cut short, keep skin between toes dry, get hard skin removed by a professional podiatrist, don't walk barefoot, especially on hot surfaces, wear wide-fitting, comfortable shoes. In general, the walking surface of the feet and the toes require a bit more love and attention than they usually get!

Figure 11.1: A summary of complications of Type 2 diabetes resulting from disorders of small blood vessels ('microvascular' complications), emphasising screening for early involvement.

177

sad sight of white sticks and guide dogs in the diabetes clinic wasn't that uncommon. In the last 10 years of my hospital clinics, I knew only a tiny number of people who had lost vision from diabetes.

Why has this welcome change occurred? Although the screening programme was important, other factors must have been involved, because visual loss from diabetes was already falling before retinal screening was up and running in England and Wales in 2008. Was it better blood glucose control? Possibly: a major clinical trial (ACCORD EYE) found that low blood glucose levels maintained for a few years did have some effect in the long term on reducing eye complications. Surprisingly, lower blood pressure didn't have any effect. This trial can't explain the overall reduction we saw across England and Wales. In truth, we don't have an explanation, but it's definitely not due to a magic silver bullet. As we'll see shortly when we discuss kidney disease, we need to get used to thinking about a medical 'portfolio', just as we do with a dietary portfolio like the Mediterranean diet. Keeping everything we can (glucose, blood pressure and cholesterol) under reasonable control certainly adds up to better outcomes in the long term (see the Steno-2 study below).

The commonest eye complication of diabetes is cataract, which occurs at an earlier age than in non-diabetic people. But treatment is just as simple and effective – day case surgery.

> **Key point:** The annual photograph detects any early problems in the retina at the back of the eye, but everyone, with or without diabetes, can develop other eye troubles. You should visit your optometrist every year for a general eye check-up.

Kidneys

Let's first recall the USA data from 1990 to 2010 shown in Chapter 9, Figure 9.1: the numbers of diabetic people requiring dialysis for kidney failure fell by 50%. I imagine the same has happened in the UK. But there is still a problem. Diabetes is no longer the commonest cause of blindness, but, in spite of the welcome decrease, it still heads the list of causes of kidney failure requiring dialysis. Fortunately, only very small numbers (about one in 1000) of Type 2s ever develop severe kidney failure – and of those, about one half get a kidney transplant. (The situation with transplants reminds us of coronary artery bypass graft operations; people with diabetes were previously not accepted for kidney transplant because it was thought they had a much higher risk of complications after surgery, including losing their new kidney through infection or rejection. That's no longer the case, and many people with both Type 1 and Type 2 diabetes now have completely successful kidney transplants.)

Estimating kidney health with blood and urine tests

But of course nobody wants to get anywhere near the point of needing a transplant. And among all the complications of Type 2 diabetes, kidney disease is very successfully prevented using a portfolio of standard diabetes treatments. Annual blood and urine tests give the best information. The blood creatinine concentration was previously the standard test of kidney function, but this has been replaced over the past few years by a measurement based on creatinine, but mathematically corrected for age, ethnicity and whether you're male or female. This is the 'eGFR' (estimated Glomerular Filtration Rate). The eGFR number reflects how well the kidneys filter impurities from the blood. Creatinine accumulates in the blood as the kidneys become less efficient, but the efficiency of filtration decreases, so as blood creatinine goes up, eGFR falls. The kidney experts have started classifying the severity of kidney disease according to eGFR. Although eGFR measurements are important, we have become a bit fixated on the precise numbers, much as we saw happening with glucose levels that define 'diabetes' or 'pre-diabetes'. Numbers always need an additional ingredient – specialist experience – to avoid the risk of raising unnecessary anxieties in people with diabetes, and this applies particularly to older people.

The other really important measurement is how much protein there is in the urine. Normally there should be none, but as diabetes begins to stress the kidneys, especially if blood pressure is high, tiny amounts of protein (albumin is the protein that's measured) leak into the urine. Previously we used urine dipstick tests, but they don't register the tiny amounts signifying early stress, so although we still use sticks as a routine test when you attend your GP or hospital for a diabetes review, there is also a laboratory urine test called ACR (albumin creatinine ratio). Because it's repeated every year, over the course of time any trends can be detected.

Using these two tests – eGFR in the blood, and ACR in the urine – we can make a reasonably accurate assessment of the state of health of the kidneys. Interestingly, the same two measurements give just as accurate a risk of heart attack as the likelihood of developing kidney failure. It's not clear why two kidney-based tests should be able to predict heart disease, but it's been known for many years. Fortunately, the treatments of both very early kidney trouble and the associated heart risk are nearly identical. We know this because of a brilliant clinical trial done at one of the most famous diabetes hospitals in the world, the Steno Institute in Denmark. Though the name of the study – Steno-2 – wasn't very exciting, the results of the study were (see References, page 231).

Key point: The results of blood and urine tests when combined give a good estimate of the risk not only of kidney disease, but of heart attacks. The risk factors for both conditions are broadly similar – blood glucose, blood pressure, cholesterol, weight and exercise.

Steno-2: Portfolio Scandinavian diabetes care

Steno-2 was a long study, running for about eight years; kidney disease takes a long time to develop. The people included were already at higher risk of kidney and heart disease because they had persistently slightly high levels of protein in the urine (elevated ACR). The idea was simple: use a portfolio of simple treatments – that is, control blood pressure, blood glucose and cholesterol, and encourage people to lose weight, stop smoking, eat healthily and exercise. Medication included a statin, low-dose aspirin and one of the blood pressure drugs that specifically target the kidneys (an ACE inhibitor or ARB; see Chapter 10). One group was supervised every few months in the hospital clinic (the 'intensive' group); the other had community care under their general practice team.

After the eight years in the study, the intensive group had lower levels of diabetic eye disease (retinopathy) and progressing kidney disease, and heart attacks were nearly 50% lower. After another five years, during which both groups were encouraged to look after themselves as well as possible (and medication was introduced as necessary in everyone who needed it), the group previously intensively treated had a 50% reduced risk of heart disease, including death from that cause. Serious eye disease requiring laser treatment was 60% lower, and only one person needed dialysis, compared with six in the group treated less intensively during the trial. After a very long follow-up period, the intensively treated group had lived on average eight years longer, mostly because they had less heart disease.

Was a huge amount of treatment needed here? And did glucose and blood pressure measurements have to be very low? Nothing of the kind. Blood pressure was good, and patients achieved the levels we currently recommend (130–140 mm). Blood glucose control using the HbA_{1c} test was 7.7% (61 mmol/mol), and cholesterol 3.8 mmol/l. These are relatively easy values to achieve in nearly everyone – and note the blood glucose level was reasonable, but not by any means low. The message is very encouraging: using relatively small amounts of well-targeted medication and attention to weight, diet and exercise, we can get remarkable results, with very low risks of severe kidney disease and a major reduction in heart attack rates.

> **Key point:** In people at higher risk of diabetic kidney complications, good blood pressure and cholesterol control with moderately good blood glucose control over a period of about eight years had a major beneficial effect on nearly every diabetic complication, not just kidney disease.

Combining moderately tough portfolio treatments together has a disproportionate effect

I apologise, but only a little, for my detailed description of the Steno-2 trial, which should have hit the headlines, but didn't. The results were remarkable, but therapy didn't involve earth-shattering drugs or technology, and the input into lifestyle wasn't especially intensive, yet complications that really matter (heart disease, eye disease and advanced kidney disease) were all reduced by an enormous amount, and life expectancy increased. A set of therapeutic portfolios – modest input into everything related to diabetes – achieved great things. Because of this the people doing the trial couldn't easily analyse if there was any *single* input that contributed the most to these good results, but their hunch was getting the cholesterol down with a statin was the most important, not, as you might imagine, reducing blood glucose levels.

Chapter 11

Neuropathy

Like kidney and eye complications, neuropathy – diabetes affecting the nerves to legs, arms and internal organs – used to have terrible outcomes, most frighteningly the loss of legs. This is another fearful complication that is much less common now, and, like all the other complications, is less frequent because Type 2 diabetes is *generally* looked after better than even 10 years ago, You understand now that controlling blood glucose levels is probably not the only aspect of treatment that has reduced neuropathy: blood pressure, cholesterol, and lifestyle (exercise, weight loss and stopping smoking) are equally important, and probably more so.

However, in people with 10 or more years of Type 2, numb toes, tingling of the feet and occasionally pain in the legs are still quite common. These symptoms, troubling though they are, don't mean that the foot or leg is threatened – but you need to be especially careful to look after your feet because the nerves relaying sensation from the feet to the brain are not fully operative, and your feet may be less sensitive, especially to heat and sharp pain. In spite of decades of research, there are no drugs that help repair nerves, but it's simple to prevent the most serious complication of neuropathy, foot ulceration.

- Ensure toenails are cut cleanly and frequently (if you can't reach or feel your feet properly get someone else to cut your nails).
- Dry thoroughly between the toes, where bacterial and fungal infections can lurk.
- If you have dry, thickened or cracked feet, moisturise with hydrating cream (for example, one of the Flexitol range).
- Never walk barefoot, especially on hot surfaces (beaches and marble floors in hot climates are a particular hazard).
- Wear well-fitting shoes (fashionistas beware – designer shoes aren't designed with diabetes in mind), and check for gravel, stones and other objects in them.

This is hardly high-tech advice but, like many of the other treatments we've discussed in Type 2 – it works.

Foot ulcers

We discussed what happens when the large blood vessels to the feet fail to carry enough blood in Chapter 9. Poor blood supply can lead to ulcers of the feet, often associated with pain, but a much more common reason for developing foot ulcers is poor sensation resulting from inefficient nerves. These ulcers usually develop in areas of the feet subjected to pressure when walking, especially under the big toe, where very high pressures occur, further increased by hard skin or callus. Podiatrists are masters at managing callus and reducing pressure on the feet, and can spot trouble very early. If you've been told your feet are at higher risk, contact your local specialist podiatrist if there are any concerning signs: skin breaks, bleeding, red skin (infection/cellulitis) or pus. Prompt X-rays, possibly including an MRI scan, then treatment with antibiotics and the use of pressure-reducing casts and footwear can usually prevent further trouble. Amputation rates aren't zero yet, but prompt and meticulous care has certainly contributed to reducing the need for surgery.

Erectile dysfunction

Erectile dysfunction (ED) is common, affecting perhaps 20 to 40% of men. It is certainly the most common complication of nerve damage in diabetes, and may overall be the commonest diabetic complication. Treatments for ED used to be uncomfortable and not very successful, but drugs such as sildenafil (Viagra) and tadalafil (Cialis) have been remarkably helpful. Treatment combinations are often used by urology specialists when simple tablet-treatments aren't fully effective.

Summary

The specific complications of diabetes caused by small vessel disease are less common, though they probably haven't decreased as spectacularly as heart attacks and strokes. The portfolio approach works for all these complications – for example, keeping blood glucose levels between 6 and 10 mmol/l, resulting in an HbA_{1c} value around 7% (53 mmol/mol), systolic blood pressure between 130 and 140, and cholesterol as low as possible. Even if it is difficult, for example, to keep the blood glucose levels to target, focus on the blood pressure and cholesterol – they are just as important as blood glucose, and in combination probably more so.

Chapter 12

Diabetes and older people

Key points

- People are living longer and developing fewer complications of Type 2 diabetes.
- Frailty is more of a risk to older Type 2s than high blood glucose levels.
- Frailty, together with obesity, is a common problem in older people: increased exercise and protein intake can improve mental and physical functioning.
- Type 2s are often given too much medication, risking severe hypoglycaemia.
- Psychological problems are common, especially depression and cognitive impairment. They need to be recognised early, and support provided early on.

People with both Type 1 and Type 2 diabetes are – fortunately – growing old gracefully and increasingly living to ripe old age in good health. Ensuring that more people can do this without troubles arising from complications, side-effects from medication and psychological difficulties are especially important considerations in older people.

Managing blood glucose in older people

Careful studies have come to the conclusion that low blood glucose levels can be more hazardous in older people than higher values (we'll discuss the numbers shortly).

One of the most dramatic and troubling cases I remember was an 80-year-old insulin-treated lady who fell against a hot radiator because her blood glucose level was low (hypoglycaemia). (She was Type 1, but hypoglycaemia – blood glucose levels under 4 mmol/l and often 3 or lower – is a significant risk in anyone taking insulin.) Because of the low blood glucose level she remained unconscious for several hours until found by her sister, by which time she had severe burns on her thighs, and needed many weeks in hospital for skin grafts. Fortunately, cases like this are extremely rare.

But there is a general message often relayed to diabetes patients: 'lower glucose is better'. In some cases, 'lower' is interpreted as not-far-off-normal, that is between 4 and 7. Major clinical studies have shown there is no advantage in going for such low levels, and of course they are associated with a greater risk of hypoglycaemia. For a variety of reasons, older people are more inclined to strive to achieve these unrealistic and potentially hazardous glucose levels.

A study of older diabetic Italian people in nursing homes found that blood glucose levels were generally rather low. There were several reasons. First, the residents weren't overweight. Although they may have had additional medical reasons for their low weight, once we pass our mid-60s, many of us experience a gradual and slow fall in weight, probably due to a declining appetite. Second, and as a result of the lower weight, many older people need less medication for blood glucose levels, though doctors find it very difficult to decrease or discontinue medication.

What blood glucose levels should older people have?

In older people generally, we should be aiming for reasonable glucose levels, for example between 7 and 11 mmol/l, but there is no harm in levels up to 15 or thereabouts in older people who are at risk of very low blood glucose levels, are frail or have dementia, and therefore might come to particular harm if they had an unexpected 'hypo'. The corresponding HbA_{1c} test of long-term control should lie somewhere between 7% (53 mmol/mol) and 8.5% (67 mmol/mol), depending on the overall health of individuals. If less medication is needed to achieve these levels, that should be seen as positive (see Chapter 7) and not in any way discriminating against the interests of older people.

When I was in hospital practice, I always promised myself that I would try and focus our conversation during a consultation not on blood glucose levels, but factors that really matter in the older person: good but not low blood pressure, the best possible cholesterol levels, and of course quality of life. But my diligent patients would generally walk in and immediately present me with a meticulous record of – their blood glucose levels – and I felt it would be deeply impolite not to start with a discussion of glucose control. However, this often meant that other more important things, such as how people and their families were managing with their diabetes overall, always got crammed into the last few minutes. It would be good if we could really change this emphasis, but I suspect it may be a while before we achieve this in practice.

Over-medication in older people

We discussed in Chapter 7 the multiple pressures on doctors to treat glucose in Type 2 to achieve lower and lower levels (the same may go for blood pressure medication – low blood pressure measurements, sometimes leading to faintness or dizziness, are often seen in older people as well as lower blood glucose levels). In short, many older people are over-medicated for diabetes. Some medications are especially liable to cause weight loss, which while desirable in the overweight and obese is much less positive in people already at not far off their expected weight. As we've seen (Chapter 7), metformin is often continued even when other drugs have been reduced or stopped, and this is because of a possibly exaggerated view of the benefit of metformin in reducing the risk of heart attacks. But metformin can suppress appetite, an effect which seems to be more common in older individuals. You can see how a vicious cycle may be set off.

The key message here is that achieving non-diabetic blood glucose measurements in older people should not, as is often the case, be a reason for congratulation. On the contrary, it should prompt a careful review of *all* medication with a view to helping restore safe values (see above for a few examples of numbers). Physicians with a specialist interest in old age are clued up about the problems associated with medication and over-medication in patients under their care, especially the need to keep doses to the absolute minimum, and also to take into account the increased risk of side-effects in older people and interactions with other medications. However, general practice teams may be less familiar with the subtlety with which medication needs to be handled in these sensitive people.

Frailty and diabetes

Over the past few years it has become clear that overall health outcomes in older people with diabetes, especially the over-80s, are not mostly determined by blood glucose levels, but much more strongly by an important and relatively new concept, termed 'frailty'. In the UK, Professor Alan Sinclair has been a powerful advocate of this radical idea, and his views, and that of other specialists in diabetes in older age, are gradually gaining acceptance.

What is 'frailty'? Like 'old age' itself, frailty is difficult to define precisely, because it encompasses so many different factors. However, two main features are the loss of muscle mass (medical term: sarcopenia) and loss of muscle function. While these factors occur in everyone who is ageing, they are more marked in people with diabetes. But they develop gradually and slowly, and may not be identified until someone has a fall. Many people are aware that they have less muscle in their legs as they get older. Most often it is men who notice this, as they have less fat on the legs than women. It's not clear why decreasing muscle mass is more prominent in people with diabetes, but we saw in Chapter 3 that in Type 2, increased fat in the liver and pancreas, which is ultimately the cause of high blood glucose levels, can also be associated with increased fat inside muscle fibres, which may contribute to increased muscle weakness.

Whatever the causes – and there is important research going on to try and uncover them – reduced muscle mass is closely linked to reduced mobility, slower walking, and less agility when faced with an uneven walking surface such as the average UK pavement. But there are more subtle consequences of frailty which show up as less agility with real-life tasks, such as housework, grocery shopping and self-care. All these have a negative impact on quality of life and increase the need for relying on others. In people with diabetes, factors that may make frailty worse include multiple medications, hypoglycaemia (of course), low blood pressure and loss of sensation in the feet (neuropathy, see Chapter 11, page 183).

Maintaining good nutrition in older people

Although frailty is increasingly recognised as a problem in older Type 2s, we don't yet have focused treatments. Trial results will emerge over the next few years. But exercise training, especially resistance exercise, and protein supplements seem to help both physical function and some components of mental functioning. Some of the physical aspects of frailty, especially those related to osteoporosis, are postponed by the Mediterranean diet. What's particularly important in older people is to encourage general good nutrition. That often means undoing some of the 'rules', including relaxing carbohydrate restriction in people who aren't overweight, because low glucose levels are much less important than overall good nutrition. It's striking how many older people with diabetes have given up simple pleasures, such as a couple of biscuits with a hot drink. In someone whose total calorie intake may already be borderline deficient, avoiding three or four biscuits a day (amounting to 240–300 kcal) may cause their weight to slide even more.

Older people also often observe the low-fat mantra, but by now we have sufficient insight into Type 2 to recognise that restricting fat – and the large amount of energy it contains – is also unwise in older people, who are in any case likely to be taking a statin. (Incidentally, older age is not associated with an increased risk of statin side-effects, but older people may be taking more medications that can interact with statins.) Any impact of a higher-fat diet on blood cholesterol is likely to be negligible, and slight weight increase in association with generally better nutrition is the most important consideration. Rigid rules, especially ones that never had a proper scientific basis in the first place, must always play a secondary role to good common sense.

> **Key point:** Older Type 2 people who are losing weight should maintain a good diet. Unnecessarily restricting carbohydrates and fats can contribute to further weight loss, muscle weakness and increased frailty.

Frailty and *obesity: a double problem in Type 2 diabetes*

Loss of muscle in the legs, leading to impaired mobility and agility, is a particular problem in older Type 2 people. But we know that Type 2 is also associated with overeating, leading to increased abdominal fat and its own associated metabolic problems. So, in later life Type 2s often have the dual problem of weaker muscles, usually not being exercised, that are expected to carry overall a greater body weight. The big tummy atop skinny legs is therefore particularly common in older people with diabetes, though the medical term (sarcopenic obesity) is perhaps a little more elegant (see Figure 12.1).

We don't have clinical trial results yet to establish what is the best lifestyle approach for people with sarcopenic obesity, but it would seem sound to cut back carbohydrates (to help reduce abdominal

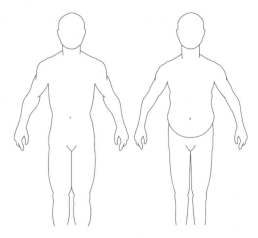

Figure 12.1: Sarcopenic obesity. The outline on the left is normal – no obesity and no sarcopenia. The typical body shape of someone with sarcopenic obesity is shown on the right. The key features are thin upper arms and thighs, and a large abdomen.

obesity and fats in the wrong places) while maintaining high protein and higher fat intake, and as much exercise as possible. In other words, try and emulate the younger bodybuilders: steak (or veg protein) and eggs with some resistance exercise. We urgently need the evidence.

Other features of ageing associated with diabetes

Other features of ageing are more common in people with diabetes than those without the condition.

Depression

Depression is known to be at least twice as common in Type 2 people. It's discussed in more detail in Chapter 13, but broadly speaking it responds well to both antidepressant medication and talking therapy. Treatment tends to improve glucose levels too, presumably as a result of people who are less depressed becoming more engaged with their diabetes.

Chapter 12

Cognitive impairment and dementia

Type 2 diabetes is associated with a slightly increased risk of dementia of both varieties, classical Alzheimer's disease and that associated with disease of the small blood vessels in the brain (vascular dementia). Some of the consequences will be obvious – for example, omitting medication and insulin, not doing blood glucose measurements or misinterpreting the results. In diabetic people with dementia, hypoglycaemia is especially common, and, hardly surprisingly, hazardous, with a high risk of falls and fractures (see below). In a large study from Germany and Austria – similar to the Italian study I mentioned before – older people with diabetes tended to have low glucose levels, but those with dementia were *more* likely to be on treatment with insulin, the drug most likely to be associated with hypoglycaemia. This demonstrates again that healthcare professionals aren't always sensitive to the best treatment for individual patients. (Just in case you're wondering, the association between insulin treatment and dementia shouldn't be taken to imply that insulin treatment *causes* dementia, or increases its risk; there's no evidence for that.)

Falls

Older people with diabetes are at particular risk of falls. Several factors are involved, including some we've already mentioned: multiple medications, muscle weakness, previous strokes (which if they are small events may not have been recognised as strokes – see Chapter 9), neuropathy (less ability to feel the feet and an additional cause of muscle weakness – see Chapter 11), blood pressure falling when standing up, and visual impairment (for example due to diabetic retinopathy, cataracts or age-related macular degeneration). Insulin treatment, especially if it results in overall low blood glucose levels (HbA$_{1c}$ under 7.0%, or 53 mmol/mol) is a risk for falls. Many of these factors can be managed positively to reduce the risk.

Social factors

Good care of Type 2 diabetes is collaborative, and often involves life partners. Illness or the death of a partner can be a terrible additional burden in managing diabetes, especially for people taking insulin. In many cases, partners have been giving injections for years, as well as monitoring blood glucose levels, and they often show wonderful skill and intuition – after all, they know their partners better than anyone. The loss of someone so dedicated to the care of diabetes can be a major blow. Hospital and general practice teams are often in a good position to identify these difficulties, though replacing the round-the-clock skills of someone who may have been helping with diabetes for decades is a huge challenge.

Summary

Maintaining 'tight' blood glucose control in old age isn't as important as in younger people, not because of elder discrimination but because it isn't as important as other diabetes-related matters – for example, maintaining meticulous blood pressure and low cholesterol levels.
In addition, the risk of small blood vessel complications (eyes, kidneys, nerves) is much lower than the spectrum of problems now called frailty. We don't have specific drugs to help frailty, but reducing medication that results in hazardously low blood glucose and blood pressure levels is a good start. In addition, older people need to maintain good nutrition with higher protein and fat intake and do as much exercise as possible to try and avoid the muscle wasting of age (sarcopenia).

Chapter 13

Psychology and Type 2 diabetes

Key points

- Managing Type 2 is as much a matter of managing the mind as medication and diet.
- Most people don't have major psychological disturbances at diagnosis, but over the following years depression and distress may become more frequent.
- Depression and Type 2 are closely linked.
- The best treatments are psychological and careful management of diabetes itself. Antidepressants don't usually help unless there are other complications present.
- The cumulative burden of managing diabetes over many years can lead to distress, and finally to burnout.
- Sympathetic and careful medical management is probably the best way of tackling diabetes distress and burnout.

Diabetes and mental health

The highly complex relationship between the mind and Type 2 diabetes has been explored over many years, but most of the research articles are concerned with depression in diabetes. Depression is common in all types of diabetes, and at all ages, and as we'll see, although it's important, it is only one of several psychological problems encountered in diabetes. One of the reasons depression has been so much of a focus is that the severity of depression can be reliably measured using carefully standardised questionnaires and interview techniques. Not very long ago, as part of their contract,

GPs in the UK were required to ask all people with diabetes to complete such a questionnaire, though I don't think anything much of practical value resulted from the exercise.

Surprisingly little is known about the range of psychological disorders that don't quite add up to depression, but which can be just as disruptive to the lives of people with Type 2. For example, 'diabetes distress', of which more shortly, is likely to cause more difficulty than full-blown depression. At the other end of the spectrum of severity, some organisations have gone so far as to consider the response to the diagnosis of Type 2 diabetes as similar to the response to a fatal diagnosis. You may know of the series of stages described by the famous psychologist, Elisabeth Kubler-Ross (denial, anger, bargaining, depression and acceptance) back in the late 1960s.

I think this is going much too far – Type 2 diabetes is hardly a fatal diagnosis after all – but Kubler-Ross's scheme covers many of the factors experienced by newly diagnosed people. In addition, there may also be a sense of guilt, and if I developed Type 2 diabetes I suspect that would be my most powerful initial feeling: I had got my comeuppance after years of 'bad' habits. Diabetes is a disorder associated with weight (though, as we have seen, most people with diabetes are no more overweight than their peers without diabetes). This then ties in with eating patterns that may be seen as abnormal, though actually they're probably no different from those of non-diabetic people either. But in my discussions with Type 2s, guilt is very common, and shows itself in all kinds of ways. For example: guilt that in some way the person has a self-inflicted condition; guilt that he/she isn't doing what he/she has been told to bring it under control (especially diet and weight loss) and guilt about the consequences of a major long-term condition on his/her family.

Psychological symptoms at the time of diagnosis

Some of the elements in Kubler-Ross's sequence are relevant when Type 2 is first diagnosed. Denial, for example, is probably present in many people with diabetes. Even if there are symptoms at the onset, they are usually due to high glucose levels (thirst, getting up in the night to go to the loo, blurred vision etc. – see Chapter 2) and don't usually last long. Do I *really* have diabetes or is it just a period of funny symptoms that have now gone away of their own accord? If there has been any weight loss it may give rise to mixed feelings: perhaps that diet we'd promised ourselves is finally working, or a little more exercise is at last having some effect rather than it being a result of poorly controlled diabetes with high blood glucose levels.

Middle-aged people who lose a lot of weight quickly and for no apparent reason may well worry that there is cancer lurking, and once that has been excluded, then there may be some – temporary – sense of relief. I think everyone has a different mix of feelings at this stage of diabetes, and that's because by the time we're in our 40s or 50s, we all have very different lives, different work and family circumstances, and a variable medical history behind us. To return to feelings of guilt, professionals need to recognise that these feelings are often present, though not often articulated, and that this is definitely not the time to compound any guilt (actually *no* time is right for that). Sadly, this still occurs, though as our understanding of the complexity of Type 2 diabetes has developed over the past 30–40 years, we fortunately see this unhelpful blame-guilt cycle much less than before.

These varied responses aren't always captured in the academic studies. Naturally, there is generally much less psychological upset when Type 2 is diagnosed than Type 1, which usually comes out of the blue in childhood, and requires massive and immediate life-changes to adapt quickly to permanent insulin treatment. But as we discussed in Chapter 2, a small number of people are first diagnosed with diabetes when they have an illness – for example, heart attack or stroke – that requires an emergency admission to hospital. I don't think these patients have ever been studied to gauge the extent of their psychological disturbance.

Stress, work and diabetes

Perhaps the most common question at diabetes onset is: 'Was it stress that brought it on?' We know that in Type 1 diabetes, medical stress – for example, a major illness or hospitalisation – is more common in the year preceding the onset of diabetes than in people who don't develop diabetes. Perhaps more interesting, major family disturbances – for example, parental separation or divorce in the previous year – also increase the risk of developing Type 1 diabetes. Type 2 is completely different. All the same, we know that some forms of stress, especially long-term stress at work, increase the risk of developing Type 2. (It also increases the risk of depression, which, as we'll see, is strongly linked to Type 2.) The key factor here may be cortisol, the major hormone released from the adrenal glands near the kidneys during psychological and physical stress. Cortisol is well known to increase insulin resistance and predispose people to developing the metabolic syndrome (see Chapter 3). We can therefore see a close biological link between stress, cortisol and the development of Type 2, and there was great interest in developing drugs that could reduce the effects of cortisol. In early trials they significantly reduced blood glucose in people with Type 2. Interestingly, adrenaline, the 'fight or flight' hormone we all know is linked to stress, probably plays no part in the development of Type 2.

> **Key point:** Long-term work stress is associated with an increased risk of developing Type 2 diabetes.

This is all very interesting, but is it of any practical value to pre-diabetic individuals or those with Type 2? There are no official studies of the effect of continuing stress at work on Type 2, but there are plenty of reasons why stressed workers might have poor blood glucose control (and for that matter, poor blood pressure control). You will see no great surprises in the list below, but have a think about factors that may operate for you and whether you can reduce them in your work life.

- Erratic meals, especially high-carbohydrate lunches wolfed down while gazing at a computer screen.
- Missing medication, especially a lunchtime dose of fast-acting insulin.
- Shift work is associated with increased risks of a range of conditions, including Type 2 diabetes, weight gain, coronary heart disease and stroke.
- Disturbed sleep patterns, associated with poor blood pressure control.
- Electronic stress – deluges of emails, in particular – is also likely to compromise blood pressure control.
- No time for work-associated activity; gym sessions postponed (see Chapter 8).

Key point: Analyse carefully what stresses you are exposed to in your workplace, and consider possible ways of reducing them.

Depression and Type 2

Since so much work has been done on Type 2 and depression, let's summarise some of the current understanding. You might think the link is relatively simple. Type 2 is a long-term condition that requires continual self-management, is associated with a range of complications, and usually needs treatment with medication that can have side-effects. So, Type 2 diabetes can *lead* to depression. But it's more complicated than that. While Type 2 is indeed associated with an increased risk of developing depressive symptoms, the converse is also true: people with depression have a higher risk of developing Type 2 diabetes. The reasons for depression leading to an increased risk of Type 2 aren't known, but stress and stress hormones, especially cortisol, may predispose to depression. It's an intriguing idea, and more research will no doubt emerge. Other hormones may be involved, including testosterone in men (and presumably abnormalities of sex hormones in females). If we take a broader view of these tentative ideas, we can see again a series of links that help us understand Type 2 diabetes as a whole-body problem, rather than as a limited condition just involving high blood glucose levels.

An even more linked-up explanation is that both Type 2 diabetes and depression share similar roots in psychosocial factors. For example, reduced activity levels, social deprivation and adverse conditions during childhood may contribute to both conditions (see Figure 13.1).

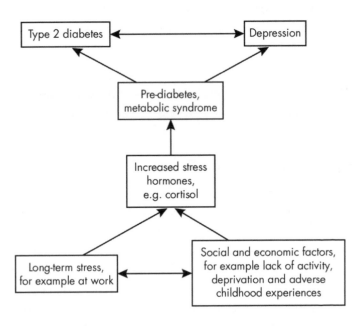

Figure 13.1: Some of the links between Type 2 diabetes, stresses during life and depression.

When depression occurs in Type 2, it is strongly associated with high blood pressure and medication for high blood pressure, being overweight, cigarette smoking, reduced physical ability to do exercise, and – most consistent of all – a greater likelihood of missing medical appointments. This last factor may well perpetuate the tendency to depression, as it is less likely to be diagnosed, intercepted and treated if people don't attend appointments. But even where medical care is very good, consultations in both hospital clinics and general practice tend to be preoccupied with blood glucose control and helping people to improve it, and a possible major underlying problem, serious depression, may not come to light.

Key point: Type 2 diabetes can lead to depression, but more intriguingly depression itself increases the risk of developing Type 2.

Treatments for depression in people with Type 2

Because diabetes and depression occur so commonly together there have been several studies to try and find effective treatments. Ideal therapy would, of course, improve symptoms of depression, but could they also improve physical function? There is some evidence for this from the Look AHEAD study (see Chapter 5 and References on page 214), where people in the intensive lifestyle group had better muscle function and were also less likely to develop depression. Frequent and intensive collaborative medical care focused on physical aspects of poorly controlled diabetes improved blood glucose, cholesterol and blood pressure and – surprisingly – also improved depression scores. In other words it looks as if intensive *medical* input improves both physical and psychological health in Type 2.

Key point: Intensive medical treatment improves measures of diabetes, including blood glucose and blood pressure, and also psychological functioning, in Type 2 people with depression.

Psychological treatments

Psychological treatments have not been as thoroughly studied as medical treatment, but all types of therapy – for example, cognitive behavioural therapy (CBT), mindfulness-based therapy, internet-based guided self-help – improve depression severity, but do not seem to improve the physical aspects of diabetes, including blood glucose control.

Antidepressants

Antidepressant medications might seem the obvious treatment, but they haven't been thoroughly investigated in long-term conditions like diabetes, and, as we've seen, psychological treatments and interventions focused on the diabetes itself are at least as effective. However, one trial found that if people choose antidepressant treatment and if symptoms improve in the first three months, then medication seems to be beneficial if it's continued. People who have both medical complications of diabetes and depression also respond well to medically orientated treatment and antidepressants. As in all areas of diabetes, the key is to select treatments that are most likely to help individuals with particular problems. Regardless of the treatment, the organisation of care – for example, how often you go for psychological treatment, and the type and dose of drug – must be properly planned and implemented and based on clinical trial protocols. A bit of extra medical input or one psychological appointment is unlikely to be of much use.

Diabetes distress

A distress response to diabetes is not a psychiatric disorder, such as depression, but is very common, perhaps occurring in nearly 50% of Type 2s. Broadly, it's the stress response (note, stress again) to living with a complex and long-term condition. Its main components won't come as a surprise:

- the demands of self-care leading to anger and frustration
- concern about an uncertain future with diabetes, and the possibility of complications
- concern about the quality of care
- perceived lack of support from family and friends.

There have been many studies on distress and its management, but in practice even those with quite severe depression may not be able to access optimum treatment, so informal management of distress falls to family, colleagues and the healthcare team. We saw that careful and attentive medical care improves depressive symptoms and standard indicators of diabetes (HbA_{1c}, blood pressure and cholesterol). Distress is often focused around practical considerations (for example, large amounts of medication, injections, excessive requirements for blood glucose testing). Doctors are often not sensitive enough to the adverse impact of people's day-to-day concerns about diabetes, nor the burden of longer-term concerns.

Diabetes burnout

Diabetes burnout is a widely used term, and very valuable. It conveys a vivid and immediate picture of someone with diabetes eventually exhausted by the stresses of maintaining 'good' glucose control, while also having to deal with family, the workplace (where the term 'burnout' originated). and the countless other day-to-day problems that compete for limited mental space. Online diabetes communities are full of discussions about this evidently common problem, but out of millions of medical articles I could only find a couple that referred to it. This itself is a significant observation: here's something that everyone is talking about electronically, yet it doesn't seem to be recognised by the medical world. We urgently need a proper definition, but until then let's think of a burnt-out person with diabetes as someone who has lived with it for a number of years, taking an ever-increasing amount of medication, perhaps who has accumulated a few complications requiring additional medical care and more frequent clinic appointments, and whose family and friends are themselves stressed with the burden of living with someone who has a long-term condition.

There are many different scenarios of burnout. I've often seen it in Type 1 and 2 people who are trying to maintain unrealistic and unhelpful 'normal' blood glucose levels; they end up doing countless finger-prick blood glucose levels and eventually, of course, become depressed and stressed by the effort and – worse – usually don't manage to achieve the unachievable. This spills over into relationship problems with friends and family, and risks further spread of conflict and anxiety. The fault here sometimes lies with healthcare professionals, who impose arbitrary blood glucose limits and then don't always support their patients to achieve them. In Type 2 I see a different variety, 'diet burnout'. Again this often results from arbitrary and unnecessary food restrictions, often of the 'you mustn't eat cake' variety. These impositions often date from many years ago, but they are alive and kicking today and perhaps even more dogmatic: think how many times you've seen internet ads for '10 foods you must [or must not] eat in order to reduce your belly fat' or similar.

One approach to burnout is to minimise practical burdens.

- Can we realistically reduce medication and excessive self-monitoring? (This was explored in Chapter 7, and discussed in relation to older people in Chapter 12.)
- Closely related: request a detailed medication review with your diabetes team or specialist pharmacist with the aim of rationalising and simplifying your drug treatment if possible. Why were they prescribed in the first place (it's often surprising that nobody – doctor or Type 2 – can remember why), and are they needed *now*? (See Chapter 7.)

These are the 'medical' approaches. Others may be needed. If you are also depressed as a result of burnout, then that needs managing as well (though, as we've seen, one of the best ways of managing depression in Type 2 is to refine the condition's medical treatment). Many people will go online for information and advice, and perhaps join a forum. It's not known how effective they are, but advice is usually sound. The small amount of irresponsible content is usually weeded out when groups of people with a shared problem are communicating with each other. Because people with Type 2 can experience a range of potentially very serious problems, some have a tendency to catastrophise – that is, imagine that they will run into a never-ending series of disabling complications. We know that any major consequences of Type 2 are not that common, and becoming less so with time, so establishing a relationship with a healthcare professional who has a realistic understanding of diabetes in the long term can be genuinely reassuring to many people.

Summary

Psychological problems are very common in Type 2 diabetes. Stress, especially at work, is a recurrent theme, and it probably increases the risk of developing Type 2. Depression also increases the risk of developing diabetes, which is less intuitive than Type 2 increasing the risk of depression. Psychological therapies are probably more effective than antidepressant medication. Again not intuitively, diabetes and depression both improve after intensive medical supervision. Diabetes distress is very common and is related in part to the practical demands of this complicated condition (for example, the medication burden).

Postscript

That wasn't too tough, was it?

In the course of this book we've gone through some difficult stuff, but now you've read *Get Tough with Type 2 Diabetes*, I hope you can begin to think about Type 2 and pre-diabetes in a slightly different way, and not as conditions caused by eating too much sugar and that can be treated just by avoiding sweet stuff in our diet and using drugs to reduce blood glucose levels. Overeating is the problem, leading to the liver and pancreas being stressed by accumulated fat, and too much carbohydrate seems to be the worst culprit. Drastically cutting down on calorie intake relieves the stress on the liver and pancreas and allows the metabolic machinery to start up again, this time more normally.

Large and small blood vessels throughout the body, but especially those supplying the heart, brain and kidneys, are damaged by Type 2, leading to heart attacks, strokes and kidney disease. We know in people without diabetes that the major contributors to these are high blood pressure, abnormal cholesterol levels and smoking – and there's no difference in Type 2 diabetes. General practitioners in the UK help Type 2s manage these very well – better than in most countries – and better blood pressure and lower cholesterol levels probably account for the large falls in heart attacks and strokes we've seen in Type 2 people in the past 15 years.

We've also learned a lot about dietary portfolios that reduce the risk of serious diabetes complications. The Mediterranean diet with lots of extra-virgin olive oil is the most dramatically effective, but reducing carbohydrates and increasing healthy protein can help with weight loss and limiting weight regain. Single superfoods or nutraceuticals may eventually turn out to contain valuable drug-like substances that reduce blood glucose levels, but there's no evidence at present that taken individually they are of any benefit. But specific portfolios help blood pressure and possibly cholesterol.

We know lots more about medical and lifestyle causes and treatments of diabetes, but it's clear that many people have psychological barriers to achieving good diabetes outcomes. Education and close medical supervision of people distressed and depressed by Type 2 are important not only for developing coping strategies but also for improving short-term outcomes, including lowering blood glucose levels and helping blood pressure.

It isn't much fun having Type 2, but we now have a much clearer picture of this very complicated condition. New knowledge and understanding are very encouraging because we can now manage Type 2 with less emphasis on drug treatment and more on self-management. Combining and balancing the two carefully, taking into account individual needs and wishes, is bound to result in better outcomes – and happier people.

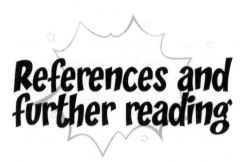

References and further reading

The key research papers and other sources of information for *Get Tough* are given below, organised by chapter. As explained in the Introduction, I have focused on sources that are 'open access' (they are free to read in full online) but on occasion papers that are behind a pay-wall are so important that I have included them also. For research papers I have cited the traditional identifiers (author names, article title, journal name etc) together with the 'DOI' – digital object identifier, which is the unique number for any online publication (many older articles do not have one) – and the 'PubMed' number which will allow you to find the 'Abstract' (summary) of any research paper on www.pubmed.gov.

How to use this book

For my discussion of the change in HbA$_{1c}$ measurements:

> Levy D. HbA$_{1c}$: changing units, changing minds – mission accomplished? *British Journal of Diabetes & Vascular Disease* 2013; 13(3): 111-114. DOI: 10.1177/1474651413495901

Chapter 1: Understanding Type 2

The 'twin cycle' hypothesis is the name given to the current thinking behind the cause of Type 2 diabetes, 'twin' referring to metabolic pathways in the liver and the pancreas. The 'twin cycle' idea is especially associated with Newcastle University and the ultra-low-calorie diet used in their pioneering studies (see Chapter 4). There are surprisingly few references suitable for non-scientists, but there are a few slides available at the following web address:

www.ncl.ac.uk/media/wwwnclacuk/
newcastlemagneticresonancecentre/files/fat-threshholds-slides.pdf
(accessed 20 December 2017).

There is a medical review paper on the twin cycle hypothesis and reversing it in the journal *Diabetic Medicine* by Professor Roy Taylor who leads the Newcastle projects:

Taylor R. Banting Memorial Lecture 2012: Reversing the twin cycles of Type 2 diabetes. *Diabetic Medicine* 2013; 30(3): 267-275. DOI: 10.1111/dme.12039. PubMed reference number 23075228. Free full text.

Chapter 2: Diagnosing diabetes

The Whitehall study in which civil servants were followed up with annual blood glucose levels. An analysis of ethnic differences found that south Asian people began their long journey towards diabetes with a slightly higher glucose level than white subjects, and the rise in the two years before diagnosis was slightly more rapid:

Hulman A, Simmons RK, Brunner EJ, Witte DR, et al. Trajectories of glycaemia, insulin sensitivity and insulin secretion in South Asian and white individuals before diagnosis of type 2 diabetes: a longitudinal analysis from the Whitehall II cohort study. *Diabetologia* 2017; 60(7): 1252-1260. doi: 10.1007/s00125-017-4275-6 PubMed reference number 23075228. Free full text.

To estimate your risk of Type 2 go to the Diabetes UK website:

Estimating your risk of diabetes. https://riskscore.diabetes.org.uk/ (accessed 20 December 2017).

Chapter 3: Pre-diabetes and the metabolic syndrome

Metabolic syndrome

There is a fully open-access journal devoted to the metabolic syndrome, the *Journal of Metabolic Syndrome*, with many links, mostly scientific, but a few of clinical interest:

> www.omicsonline.org/ArchiveJMS/articleinpress-metabolic-syndrome-open-access.php (accessed 20 December 2017).

The argument/discussion about the 'definition' of the metabolic syndrome has been rumbling on for years. It is mostly concerned with 'cut off points' for glucose, blood pressure, waist measurements and lipid values as these are the easily measurable characteristics of the syndrome. The International Diabetes Federation issued their most recent document in 2014:

> IDF (2006) The IDF consensus worldwide definition of the Metabolic Syndrome. www.idf.org/e-library/consensus-statements/60-idfconsensus-worldwide-definitionof-the-metabolic-syndrome.html (accessed 21 December 2017).

Progression from pre-diabetes to diabetes

There have been various clinical trials, mostly from the 1980s–2000s, that attempted to reduce the risk of progression from pre-diabetic blood glucose levels to diabetes itself. In particular:

- The Diabetes Prevention Program (USA), which used lifestyle in one group and metformin in another:

> Diabetes Prevention Program Research Group. Reduction in the incidence of type 2 diabetes with lifestyle intervention or metformin. *New England Journal of Medicine* 2002; 346(6): 393-403. DOI: 10.1056/NEJMoa012512 PubMed reference number: 11832527. Free full text.

- The important Da Qing study in Chinese people, using weight loss, exercise, or both, showing that all these interventions are effective:

  Pan XR, Li GW, Hu YH, Yang WY, et al. Effects of diet and exercise in preventing NIDDM in people with impaired glucose tolerance. The Da Qing IGT and Diabetes Study. *Diabetes Care* 1997; 20(4): 537-544. PubMed reference number: 9096977. Only the short abstract (summary of the study) is available online, not the full paper.

- The remarkable follow-up of the Da Qing study, showing reduction in cardiovascular events 23 years after the initial lifestyle interventions:

  Li G, Zhang P, Wang J, An Y, et al. Cardiovascular mortality, all-cause mortality, and diabetes incidence after lifestyle intervention for people with impaired glucose tolerance in the Da Qing Diabetes Prevention Study: a 23-year follow-up study. *Lancet Diabetes Endocrinology* 2014; 2(6): 474-480. DOI: 10.1016/S2213-8587(14)70057-9. PubMed reference number: 24731674. Again, only the short abstract is available online.

- The Finnish Diabetes Prevention Study investigated lifestyle intervention (average achieved weight loss 4 kg (9 lb), and increased activity) in very overweight people with pre-diabetes (average BMI 31). Progression to diabetes was reduced by nearly 60%:

  Tuomilehto J, Lindstrom J, Eriksson JG, Valle TT, et al. Prevention of type 2 diabetes mellitus by changes in lifestyle among subjects with impaired glucose tolerance. *New England Journal of Medicine* 2001; 344: 1343-1350. DOI: 10.1056/ NEJM200105033441801. PubMed reference number: 11333990. Free full text.

Non-alcoholic fatty liver disease:

For more on treatment I suggest:

> Hsu WF, S LY, Lin HJ, Chang HH. A review of western
> and traditional Chinese medical approaches to managing
> nonalcoholic fatty liver disease. *Evidence Based Complementary
> and Alternative Medicine* 2016, Article ID 6491420, 12 pages.
> DOI.org/10.1155/2016/6491420. PubMed reference number:
> 27872651. Free full text.

Polycystic ovary syndrome (PCOS)

A scientific review of complementary treatments, concluded, like they
nearly all have to for nearly every condition, that there is suggestive
evidence for benefit, but not yet supported by sufficiently rigorous
clinical trials:

> Arentz S, Smith CA, Abbott J, Bensoussan A. Nutritional
> supplements and herbal medicines for women with polycystic
> ovary syndrome; a systematic review and meta-analysis. *BMC
> Complementary and Alternative Medicine* 2017; 17(1): 500.
> DOI: 10.1186/s12906-017-2011-x. PubMed reference number:
> 29178904. Free full text.

Obstructive sleep apnoea

For the effect of CPAP treatment on cardiovascular outcomes in
people with obstructive sleep apnoea see:

> McEvoy RD, Antic NA, Heeley E, Luo Y, et al. CPAP for
> prevention of cardiovascular events in obstructive sleep apnea.
> *New England Journal of Medicine* 2016; 375: 919-931. DOI:
> 10.1056/NEJMoa1606599. PMID Reference number: 27571048.
> Free full text.

Gout

There is very little scientific literature on non-drug treatment of gout, and this in part reflects the very effective medication available. This is an article written for general practitioners in the USA:

> Hainer BL, Matheson E, Wilkes RT. Diagnosis, treatment, and prevention of gout. *American Family Physician* 2014; 90(12): 831-836. PubMed reference number: 25591183.

Chapter 4: Is Type 2 potentially reversible?

The Newcastle research

The original research paper on the Newcastle approach to Type 2 was published in 2011. It is known as The Counterbalance study (COUNTERacting BetA cell failure by Long term Action to Normalise Calorie intakE):

> Lim EL, Hollingsworth KG, Aribisala BS, Chen MJ, Mathers JC, Taylor R. Reversal of type 2 diabetes: normalisation of beta cell function in association with decreased pancreas and liver triacylglycerol. *Diabetologia* 2011; 54(10): 2506-2514. DOI: 10.1007/s00125-011-2204-7 PubMed reference number: 21656330. Free full text.

The follow-up paper using the same dietary approach in people with both short- and long-duration diabetes was published in 2016:

> Stevens S, Hollingsworth KG, Al-Mrabeth A, Avery L, et al. Very low-calorie diet and 6 months of weight stability in Type 2 diabetes: pathophysiological changes in responders and nonresponders. *Diabetes Care* 2016; 39(5): 808-815. DOI: 10.2337/dc15-1942. PubMed reference number: 27002059 (abstract only, not full text).

The DiRECT study

The DiRECT study, which reported extending this initially experimental approach to a much larger group of Type 2s, was published in 2017:

> Lean MEJ, Leslie WS, Barnes AC, Brosnahan N, et al. Primary care-led weight management for remission of type 2 diabetes (DiRECT): an open-label, cluster-randomised trial. *Lancet* 2018; 391(10120):541-551. DOI: org/10.1016/S0140-6736(17)33102-1. PubMed reference number: 29221645 (abstract only).

The United Kingdom Prospective Diabetes Study (UKPDS)

There are no easily available full-text reports of the UKPDS, but there is a valuable website of the Oxford research unit where the UKPDS (and many other studies) have been carried out:

> www.dtu.ox.ac.uk/UKPDS/ (accessed 28 December 2017).

Chapter 5: Taking control of calories

The Look AHEAD study

The reference for this study is:

> The Look AHEAD Reaearch Group. Cardiovascular effects of intensive lifestyle intervention in type 2 diabetes. *New England Journal of Medicine* 2013; 369: 145-154. DOI: 10.1056/ NEJMoa1212914 PubMed reference number: 23796131. Free full text.

ACCORD, ADVANCE and VADT trials

This trio of major trials was published between 2008 and 2010. These studies were designed after UKPDS reported its main results in 1998. In UKPDS, reducing average blood glucose levels over several years from about 8% (64 mmol/mol) to 7% (53 mmol/mol) slightly reduced the risk of a heart attack. The following trials attempted to find out whether this effect was consistent. Participants were large groups of Type 2 people in their 60s, with about 10 years of diabetes, many of whom had evidence of a previous stroke or heart disease, so they were at higher risk of another event. In each trial, one group was given intensive education and treatment to reduce overall glucose levels, while the other group was given more routine levels of care. They continued for between 6 and 10 years. Broadly, they showed that improved glucose control – in some cases near-normal glucose values – had no meaningful effect on reducing these diabetic complications (one, ACCORD, detected increased harm in the intensively treated people who were often taking multiple glucose-lowering medications). Some showed a slight benefit in kidney disease. After very long-term follow-up there were detectable but small reductions in heart attack rates. The results of these very important trials never really made the headlines, perhaps in part because they didn't support the idea that very low glucose levels improved long-term complications. But this shouldn't be a surprise: Type 2 is much more than just high blood glucose control. More surprising were the additional findings that lowering blood pressure and intensifying cholesterol treatment also didn't have major effects on complications.

The reference for the ACCORD study is:

The ACCORD Study Group. Effects of intensive glucose lowering in type 2 diabetes *New England Journal of Medicine* 2008; 358: 2545-2559. DOI: 10.1056/NEJMoa0802743. PubMed reference number: 18539917. Free full text.

The reference for the long-term ACCORD follow-up study is:

The ACCORD Study Group. Long-term effects of intensive glucose lowering on cardiovascular outcomes. *New England Journal of Medicine* 2011; 364: 818-828. DOI: 10.1056/NEJMoa1006524. PubMed reference number: 21366473. Free full text.

The reference for the ADVANCE study is:

ADVANCE Collaborative Group. Intensive blood glucose control and vascular outcomes in patients with type 2 diabetes. *New England Journal of Medicine* 2008; 358(24): 2560-2572. DOI: 10.1056/NEJMoa0802987. PubMed reference number: 18539916. Free full text.

The reference for the long-term follow-up is:

Zoungas S, Chalmers J, Neal B, Billot L, et al. Follow-up of blood-pressure lowering and glucose control in type 2 diabetes. *New England Journal of Medicine* 2014; 371: 1392-1406. DOI: 10.1056/NEJMoa1407963. PubMed reference number: 25234206. Free full text.

The reference for the VADT study is:

Duckworth W, Abraira C, Moritz T, Reda D, et al. Glucose control and vascular complications in veterans with type 2 diabetes. *New England Journal of Medicine* 2009; 360: 129-139. DOI: 10.1056/NEJMoa0808431. PubMed reference number: 19092145. Free full text.

Steno-2 study

This is a famous multimodal interventional study (medication and lifestyle) in Danish Type 2 people with minor kidney involvement caused by diabetes. Below is the reference to the most recent report, showing that the intensively treated patient group had fewer heart attacks, fewer overall diabetes complications and longer life expectancy. Blood glucose control was not especially good (HbA$_{1c}$ 7.7%, 61 mmol/mol): the portfolio approach works well.

Gaede P, Oellgaard J, Carstensen B, Rossing P, et al. Years of life gained by multifactorial intervention in patients with type 2 diabetes mellitus and microalbuminuria: 21 years follow-up on the Steno-2 randomised trial. *Diabetologia* 2016; 59(11): 2298-2307. DOI: 10.1007/s00125-016-4065-6. PubMed reference number: 27531506. Free full text.

Diet studies

The following references all relate to studies of diet discussed within the chapter.
DIOGENES:

Larsen TM, Dalskov SM, van Baak M, Papdaki A, et al: Diet, Obesity and Genese (Diogenes) Project. Diets with high or low protein content and glycemic index for weight-loss maintenance. *New England Journal of Medicine* 2010; 363(22): 2102-2113. DOI: 10.1056/NEJMoa1007137. PubMed reference number: 21105792. Free full text.

DiRECT trial:

Shai I, Schwarzfuchs D, Henkin Y, Shahar DR, et al: DiRECT group. Weight loss with a low-carbohydrate, Mediterranean, or low-fat diet. *New England Journal of Medicine* 2008; 359: 229-241. DOI: 10.1056/NEJMoa0708681. PubMed reference number: 18635428. Free full text.

Lyon Diet Heart study:

de Lorgeril M, Salen P, Martin J-L, Monjaud I, Delaye J, Mamelle N. Mediterranean diet, traditional risk factors, and the rate of cardiovascular complications after myocardial infarction: final report of the Lyon Diet Heart Study. *Circulation* 1999; 99: 779-785. DOI: org/10.1161/01.CIR.99.6.779. PubMed reference number: 9989963. Free full text.

PREDIMED study:

Estruch R, Ros E, Salas-Salvado J, Covas M-I, et al. Primary prevention of cardiovascular disease with a Mediterranean diet. *New England Journal of Medicine* 2013; 368: 1279-1290. DOI: 10.1056/NEJMoa1200303. PubMed reference number: 23432189. Free full text.

Mediterranean diet in Greece:

Trichopoulou A, Costacou T, Bamia C, Trichopoulos D. Adherence to a Mediterranean diet and survival in a Greek population. *New England Journal of Medicine* 2003; 348(26): 2599-2608. DOI: 10.1056/NEJMoa025039. PubMed reference number: 12826634. Free full text.

Low glycaemic index carbohydrates in Type 2 diabetes:

Wolever TM, Gibbs AL, Mehling C, Chiasson JL, et al. The Canadian Trial of Carbohydrates in Diabetes (CCD), a 1-y controlled trial of low-glycemic-index dietary carbohydrate in type 2 diabetes: no effect on glycated haemoglobin but reduction in C-reactive protein. *American Journal of Clinical Nutrition* 2008; 87(1): 114-125. PubMed Reference number: 18175744. Free full text.

Carbohydrates, saturated fat and cardiovascular disease (PURE study):

Dehghan M, Mente A, Zhang X, Swiminathan S, et al. Associations of fats and carbohydrate intake with cardiovascular disease and mortality in 18 countries from five continents (PURE): a prospective cohort study. *Lancet* 2017; 390(10107): 2050-2062. DOI: http://dx.doi.org/10.1016/S0140-6736(17)32252-3. PubMed reference number: 28864332. Abstract only.

A relatively new concept is 'ultra-processed' food, which has recently been identified as a serious risk factor for obesity in the population in general, and very likely for Type 2 as well. Ultra-processed foods are pre-packaged and made mostly from artificial products, often with only a small proportion of ingredients that you could buy or prepare yourself. Examples include carbonated drinks, mass-produced packaged breads and buns, margarines, cakes, breakfast cereals and energy bars, energy and milk drinks, fruit yoghurts and drinks, and many ready-to-heat products, including pies, pasta and pizzas, burgers and instant soups. In a 2018 report, about 50% of food in UK households was ultra-processed – the highest proportion out of 19 European countries. In Mediterranean countries the proportion was much lower – for example, 10% in Portugal, 13% in Italy and 14% in France. This is another powerful endorsement of the benefits of the home-cooked Mediterranean diet.

Monteiro CA, Moubarac JC, Levy RB, Canella DS, Louzada MLDC, Cannon G. Household availability of ultra-processed foods and obesity in nineteen European countries. *Public Health Nutrition* 2018; 21(1): 18-26. DOI: 10. 1017/ S1368980017001379. PubMed reference number: 28714422. Abstract only.

Book/website

The following book provides an astonishingly simple and effective pictorial way of estimating the calorie, fat and carbohydrate content of thousands of foods and food products, taking into account portion size:

Cheyette C, Balolia Y. *Carbs & Cals: Carb & Calorie Counter.* 6th ed. London: Chello Publishing; 2016.

Chapter 6: 'Superfoods' and nutraceuticals

Assessments of nutraceuticals

There is an authoritative website sponsored by a division of the

National Institutes of Health in the USA – the Office of Dietary Supplements. Every supplement has a full article which summarises all the evidence on a particular food or supplement, and draws some conclusions on its potential clinical value. Although the website is intended for professionals, it is well written and easy to understand. Because it's limited to assessing available evidence, you'll understand this is not the site to go to if you want to find hype on the latest superfood:

https://ods.od.nih.gov/factsheets (accessed 31 December 2017).

WebMD is also a reliable source:

www.WebMD.com (accessed 31 December 2017).

Individual nutraceuticals

Chromium

This is a careful recent study. Chromium nicotinate taken for three months had no effect on several important measurements in Type 2 diabetes (glucose, insulin effectiveness, weight, waist measurement):

Guimaraes MM, Carvalho AC, Silva MS. Effect of chromium supplementation on the glucose homeostasis and anthropometry of type 2 diabetic patients. *Journal of Trace Elements in Medicine and Biology* 2016; 36: 65-72. DOI: 10.1016/j.jtemb.2016.04.002 PubMed reference number: 27259354. Abstract only.

Cocoa

The website of the COSMOS trial of cocoa supplements (COcoa Supplement and Multivitamin Outcomes Study (COSMOS) is:

www.cosmostrial.org/ (accessed 24 December 2017).

Resveratrol

There is good evidence that resveratrol does not improve metabolic health in Type 2 diabetes:

Timmers S, de Ligt M, van de Weijer T, Hansen J, et al. Resveratrol as add-on therapy in subjects with well-controlled type 2 diabetes: a randomized controlled trial. *Diabetes Care* 2016; 39(12): 2211-2217. DOI: 10.2337/dc16-0499. PubMed reference number: 27852684. Abstract only.

Vinegar taken with meals

In most, but not all, studies, vinegar taken with high-glycaemic index foods reduces the blood glucose level after the meal. This is a neat and well-conducted study:

Liatis S, Grammatikou S, Poulia KA, et al. Vinegar decreases postprandial hyperglycemia in patients with type II diabetes when added to a high, but not to a low, glycemic index meal. *European Journal of Clinical Nutrition* 2010; 64(7): 727-732. DOI: 10.1038/ejcn.2010.89. PubMed reference number: 20502468. Abstract only.

Chapter 7: Keeping your medication to a minimum

Lifestyle

Intensive lifestyle intervention and drug treatment can be equally beneficial in reducing blood pressure – a comparison of Look AHEAD (lifestyle) and ACCORD (drug treatment):

Espeland MA, Probstfield J, Hire D, Redmon JB, et al. Systolic blood pressure control among individuals with type 2 diabetes: a comparative effectiveness analysis of three interventions. *American Journal of Hypertension* 2015; 28(8): 995-1009. DOI: 10.1093/ajh/hpu292. PubMed reference number: 25666468. Free full text.

DASH

For the DASH diet for hypertension see:

www.dashdiet.org (accessed 31 December 2017).

This is the report of the original DASH study (1997):

Appel LJ, Moore TJ, Obarzanek E, Vollmer WM, et al. A clinical trial of the effects of dietary patterns on blood pressure. DASH Collaborative Research Group. *New England Journal of Medicine*1997; 336(16): 117-1124. PubMed reference number: 9099655. Free full text.

Nutraceuticals

This is a general review of their role in the prevention of vascular disease:

Sosnowska B, Penson P, Banach M. The role of nutraceuticals in the prevention of cardiovascular disease *Cardiovascular Diagnosis and Therapy* 2017; 7(Suppl 1): S21-S31. DOI: 10.21037/cdt.2017.03.20. PubMed reference number: 28529919. Free full text.

For nutraceuticals in the treatment of high cholesterol see:

Nutraceuticals in hypercholesterolaemia: an overview (*British Journal of Pharmacology*, 2017). PubMed reference number: 27685833. Free full text.

Salt

The science is established – too much salt is strongly associated with a higher risk of cardiovascular diseases – but the politics rumble on. This is a recent paper published in a journal of public health:

Reeve B, Magnusson R. Reprint of: food reformulation and the (neo)-liberal state: new strategies for strengthening voluntary salt

reduction programs in the UK and USA. *Public Health* 2015;
129(8): 1061-1073. DOI: 10.1016/j.puhe.2015.04.021. PubMed
reference number: 26027448. Free full text.

Chapter 8: Activity and exercise

The World Health Organization web address where you can find
their recommendations on activity levels for good health is:

www.who.int/topics/physical_activity/en/ (accessed 26 December
2017).

If you're curious how many METs you expend raking your lawn
(4.0) or playing guitar (standing) in your rock and roll band (3.0) –
since you ask, the same as juggling – this is the super-official list:

http://prevention.sph.sc.edu/tools/docs/documents_compendium.
pdf (accessed 26 December 2017)

Activity levels assessed at the beginning of the ADVANCE trial
(see Chapter 5) and diabetes-related outcomes after an average
follow-up of eight years are reported here:

Blomster JI, Chow CK, Zoungas S, Woodward M, et al. The
influence of physical activity on vascular complications and
mortality in patients with type 2 diabetes mellitus. *Diabetes
Obesity and Metabolism* 2013; 15(11): 1008-1012. DOI:
10.1111/dom.12122. PubMed reference number: 23675676.
Abstract only.

Reducing medication with exercise: a careful trial in Denmark,
focusing on exercise (around six weekly aerobic sessions of 30–60
minutes, combined with anaerobic exercise in two or three of the
sessions). Patients already had very good blood glucose control
(average HbA_{1c} 6.7%), so no meaningful improvements could be
expected, but nearly three-quarters of the intensive lifestyle group

reduced their diabetes medication, compared with only one-quarter of the group given routine care:

> Johansen MY, MacDonald CS, Hansen KB, Karstoft K, et al. Effect of an intensive lifestyle intervention on glycemic control in patients with type 2 diabetes: a randomized clinical trial. *Journal of the American Medical Association* 2017; 18(7): 637-649. DOI: 10.1001/jama.2017.10169. PubMed reference number: 28810024. Abstract only.

Technology and exercise

Fitbits don't increase physical activity in Singapore ...

> Finkelstein EA, Haaland BA, Bilger M, Sahasranaman A, et al. Effectiveness of activity trackers with and without incentives to increase physical activity (TRIPPA): a randomised controlled trial. *Lancet Diabetes and Endocrinology* 2016; 4(12): 983-995. DOI: 10.1016/S2213-8587(16)30284-4. PubMed reference number: 27717766. Abstract only.

... or in Canadian university students:

> Sharp P, Caperchione C. The effects of a pedometer-based intervention on first-year university students: a randomized control trial. *Journal of the American College of Health* 2016; 64(8): 630-638. DOI: 10.1080/07448481.2016.1217538. PubMed reference number: 27471879. Abstract only.

The benefits of intermittent and high-intensity exercise

Looking at the effect of intermittent exercise during an otherwise sedentary day – for example, at work – the following paper describes the beneficial effects of walking for about six minutes every hour on insulin and glucose levels in non-diabetic people. Standing up didn't carry the same benefits:

Pulsford RM, Blackwell J, Hillsdon M, Kos K. Intermittent walking, but not standing, improves postprandial insulin and glucose relative to sustained sitting: a randomised cross-over study in inactive middle-aged men. *Journal of Science and Medicine in Sport* 2017; 20(3): 278-283. DOI: 10.1016/j.jsams.2016.08.012. PubMed reference number: 27633397. Abstract only.

Intermittent high intensity training improves heart function and structure, and reduces liver fat (by about 40%) in Type 2s. The study was done by the same Newcastle group who taught us about remission in Type 2 with very low-calorie diets:

Cassidy S, Thoma C, Hallsworth K, Parikh J, et al. High intensity intermittent exercise improves cardiac structure and function and reduces liver fat in patients with type 2 diabetes: a randomised controlled trial *Diabetologia* 2016; 59(1): 56-66. DOI: 10.1007/s00125-015-3741-2. PubMed reference number: 26350611. Free full text.

Chapter 9: Looking after your heart and arteries

Overall changes in risk

Reduction in major complications of Type 2 diabetes in the USA over the past 20 years are described here:

Gregg EW, Li Y, Wang J, Burrows NR, et al. Changes in diabetes-related complications in the United States, 1990–2010 *New England Journal of Medicine* 2014; 370(16): 1514-1523. DOI: 10.1056/NEJMoa1310799. PubMed reference number: 24738668. Free full access.

Heart disease in south Asian people

The first research paper shows that younger south Asians with heart disease now live longer than their white UK counterparts, indicating huge improvements in medical care and self-management over a relatively short period:

> Wright AK, Kontopantelis E, Emsley R, Buchan I, et al. Life expectancy and cause-specific mortality in type 2 diabetes: a population-based cohort study quantifying relationships in ethnic subgroups. *Diabetes Care* 2017; 40(3): 338-345. DOI: 10.2337/dc16-1616. PubMed reference number: 27998911. Abstract only.

The second isn't strictly related to heart disease but is a good reminder of the value of evidence over opinion. When exercise is measured objectively, south Asian people do as much as white UK people, but when asked to estimate their activity levels, don't exaggerate as much (see also Chapter 8):

> Yates T, Henson J, Edwardson C, Bodicoat DH, Davies MJ, Khunti K. Differences in levels of physical activity between white and south Asian populations within a healthcare setting: impact of measurement type in a cross-sectional study. *BMJ Open* 2015; 5(7): e006181. DOI: 10.1136/bmjopen-2014-006181. PubMed reference number: 26204908. Free full text.

Risk reduction associated with interventions

In people with stable coronary artery disease involving two arteries, very intensive lifestyle management was equally effective compared with placing stents. This is the report of one of these studies, COURAGE:

> Sedlis SP, Hartigan PM, Teo KK, Maron DJ, et al. Effect of PCI [percutaneous coronary intervention, that is stent placement] on long-term survival in patients with stable ischemic heart disease. *New England Journal of Medicine* 2015; 373(20): 1937-1946. DOI: 10.1056/NEJMoa1505532. PubMed reference number: 26559572. Free full text.

Intensive cardiac rehabilitation reduces the risk of further cardiac events and increases life expectancy:

> Bittner V, Bertolet M, Barraza FR, Farkouh ME, et al (BARI 2D Study Group). Comprehensive cardiovascular risk factor control improves survival. *Journal of the American College of Cardiology* 2015; 66(7): 765-773. DOI: 10.1016/j. jacc.2015.06.019. PubMed reference number: 26271057. Free full text.

Using sophisticated cardiac screening tests to identify people with 'silent' coronary artery disease has not been shown to improve cardiac outcomes compared with people who had prompt access to the appropriate tests as soon as they developed symptoms. This is the report of one such trial, DIAD:

> Young LH, Wackers FJ, Chyun DA, Davey JA, et al. Cardiac outcomes after screening for asymptomatic coronary artery disease in patients with type 2 diabetes: the DIAD study: a randomized controlled trial *Journal of the American Medical Association* 2009; 301(15): 1547-1555. DOI: 10.1001/ jama.2009.476. PubMed reference number: 19366774. Free full text.

Website

Self-assess your risk of developing heart disease. The huge UK QRISK database is regularly updated and is now in its third version (QRISK3):

> https://qrisk.org/three/ (accessed 31 December 2017).

Chapter 10: Blood pressure and cholesterol

Hypertension

A list of blood pressure monitors recommended by the British

Hypertension Society for use at home can be found here:

http://bhsoc.org/bp-monitors/bp-monitors/ (accessed 28 December 2017).

The importance of taking blood pressure treatment regularly (= 'good/high adherence') is supported by this study:

Kim S, Shin DW, Yun JM, Hwang Y, et al. Medication adherence and the risk of cardiovascular mortality and hospitalization among patients with newly prescribed antihypertensive medication. *Hypertension* 2016; 67(3): 506-512. DOI: 10.1161/ HYPERTENSIONAHA.115.06731. PubMed reference number: 26865198. Abstract only.

Treatment of resistant hypertension has been studied extensively. This is one of a series of sophisticated clinical trials from the UK (the PATHWAY studies) that have used scientific understanding of hypertension to combine older antihypertensive drugs in clever new ways. The results are impressive, and have really helped people previously taking large bundles of blood pressure treatments, and often developing side-effects on them, with little impact on their blood pressure. (And they also feel much better with the new treatments.) This is another example of the real benefits of 'thinking' medicine:

Brown MJ, Williams B, Morant SV, Webb DJ, et al. Effect of amiloride, or amiloride plus hydrochlorothiazide, versus hydrochlorothiazide on glucose tolerance and blood pressure (PATHWAY-3): a parallel-group, double-blind randomised phase 4 trial. *Lancet Diabetes and Endocrinology* 2016; 4(2): 136-147. DOI: 10.1016/S2213-8587(15)00377-0. PubMed reference number: 26489809. Free full text.

Cholesterol

The CARDS study was the first statin trial conducted in an otherwise well group of Type 2s without known heart disease or stroke:

Colhoun HM, Betteridge DJ, Durrington PN, Hitman GA, et al. Primary prevention of cardiovascular disease with atorvastatin in type 2 diabetes in the Collaborative Atorvastatin Diabetes Study (CARDS): multicentre randomised placebo-controlled trial. *Lancet* 2004; 364(9435): 685-696. DOI: 10.1016/S0140-6736(04)16895-5. PubMed reference number: 15325833. (Abstract only. Sadly, 14 years after CARDS was published, the study is still not available in free full text form)

Negative media stories about statins

The evidence from Denmark is clear – after negative media stories about statins, some people discontinue taking statin treatment. Those with known heart disease are less likely to discontinue, but those with other blood vessel disorders and high blood pressure are more likely to discontinue:

Kriegbaum M, Liisberg KB, Wallach-Kildemoes H. Pattern of statin use changes following media coverage of its side effects *Patient Preference and Adherence* 2017; 11: 1151-1157. DOI: 10.2147/PPA.S133168. PubMed reference number: 28744105. Free full text.

Nielsen SF, Nordestgaard BG. Negative statin-related news stories decrease statin persistence and increase myocardial infarction and cardiovascular mortality: a nationwide prospective cohort study. *European Heart Journal* 2016; 37(11): 908-916. DOI: 10.1093/eurheartj/ehv641. PubMed reference number: 26643266. Free full text.

Alternatives to statins

Apart from the very new injectable PCSK9 agents, ezetimibe is the only non-statin agent shown in clinical trials to reduce the risk of vascular events:

> Cannon CP, Blazing MA, Giugliano RP, McCagg A, et al. Ezetimibe added to statin therapy after acute coronary syndromes. *New England Journal of Medicine* 2015; 372(25): 2387-2397. DOI: 10.1056/NEJMoa1410489. PubMed reference number: 26039521. Free full text.

Chapter 11: Avoiding eye, kidney and nerve complications

Diabetic eye disease (retinopathy)

The ACCORD study found that very intensive blood glucose control tended to slow any progression of diabetic eye disease, but it required very low blood glucose levels (e.g. HbA_{1c} 6.0% or lower (42 mmol/mol)) that carried risks associated with hypoglycaemia. Interestingly, very good blood pressure control didn't reduce progression. The whole portfolio (lifestyle and judicious medication) is probably more important than individual treatments:

> ACCORDION Study Group. Persistent effects of intensive glycemic control on retinopathy in type 2 diabetes on the Action to Control Cardiovascular Risk in Diabetes (ACCORD) follow-on study. *Diabetes Care* 2016; 39(7): 1089-1100. DOI: 10.2337/dc16-0024. PubMed reference number: 27289122. Free full text.

General review of diabetic eye disease, focusing on a relatively new group of drugs, the anti-VEGF agents, which are of real value in stabilising visual function in a form of retinopathy specifically associated with Type 2 diabetes known as maculopathy or macular oedema, and which used to be treated with laser. They are also of great value in some forms of age-related macular degeneration (AMD), a very common cause of poor vision in older people. Although it is not associated with high blood glucose levels, AMD patients often have other insulin-resistant characteristics. These drugs were originally used (and still are) in cancer chemotherapy, where they reduce abnormal blood vessels in tumours. Only minute doses are needed in eye disease:

Stewart MW. Treatment of diabetic retinopathy: Recent advances and unresolved challenges *World Journal of Diabetes* 2016; 7(16): 333-341. DOI: 10.4239/wjd.v7.i16.333. PubMed reference number: 27625747. Free full text.

Diabetic kidney disease

This is the reference for the final report of the Steno-2 study which showed that eight years of careful treatment of risk factors for kidney disease not only reduced the risk of kidney failure and heart attacks but bought extra years of life:

Gaede P, Oellgaard J, Carstensen B, Rossing P, et al. Years of life gained by multifactorial intervention in patients with type 2 diabetes mellitus and microalbuminuria: 21 years follow-up on the Steno-2 randomised trial *Diabetologia* 2016; 59(11): 2298-2307. DOI: 10.1007/s00125-016-4065-6. PubMed reference number: 27531506. Free full text.

Chapter 12: Diabetes and older people

Hypoglycaemia in older Type 2s

Older Italian people had generally low blood glucose levels, and those taking sulfonylurea medication, the tablets associated with the highest risk of hypoglycaemia, were less adept at managing their everyday lives:

Abbetecola AM, Bo M, Armellini F, D'Amico F, et al. Tighter glycemic control is associated with ADL [activities of daily living] physical dependency losses in older adults using sulfonylureas or miglitinides: results from the DIMORA study. *Metabolism* 2015. PubMed reference number: 26318195. Abstract only.

Frailty and diabetes

The following is a review article by Professor Alan Sinclair and his colleagues, who pioneered clinical research on diabetes in the elderly. His view is that ideal blood glucose levels in frail elderly people should be more than 6 mmol/l and less than 15:

Abdelhafiz AH, Koay L, Sinclair AJ. The effect of frailty should be considered in the management plan of older people with type 2 diabetes. *Future Science OA* 2016; 2(1): FSO102. DOI: 10.4155/fsoa-2015-0016. PubMed reference number 28031949. Free full text.

Over-treatment

Dementia, diabetes and hypoglycaemia – a particularly hazardous trio – were made worse in this German/Austrian study by an increased tendency of Type 2s with cognitive impairment to be treated with insulin, the drug by far the most likely to cause hypoglycaemia:

Prinz N, Stingl J, Dapp A, Denkinger MD, et al. High rate of hypoglycemia in 6770 type 2 patients with comorbid dementia: a multicentre cohort study on 215,932 patients from the German/Austrian diabetes registry. *Diabetes Research and Clinic Practice* 2016; 112: 73-81. DOI: 10.1016/j.diabres.2015.10.026. PubMed reference number: 26563590. Abstract only.

Website

Diabetes Frail is the UK organisation specifically devoted to research and best clinical practice in older people with diabetes:

www.diabetesfrail.org (accessed 31 December 2017).

Chapter 13: Psychology and Type 2 diabetes

The relationship between short sleep times and high blood pressure during the night was shown in this study:

Yang H, Haack M, Gautam S, Meier-Ewert HK, Mullington JM. Repetitive exposure to shortened sleep leads to blunted sleep-associated blood pressure dipping. *Journal of Hypertension* 2017; 35(6): 1187-1194. DOI: 10.1097/HJH.0000000000001284. PubMed reference number: 28169885. Abstract only.

Job burnout is a significant risk factor for a wide variety of serious medical and psychological conditions, including Type 2 diabetes:

Salvagioni DAJ, Melanda FN, Mesas AE, Gonzalez AD, Gabani FL, Andrade SM. Physical, psychological and occupational consequences of job burnout: a systematic review of prospective studies. *PLoS One* 2017; 12(10): e0185781. DOI: 10.1371/journal.pone.0185781. PubMed reference number: 28977041. Free full text.

Depression

Intensive lifestyle intervention in the Look AHEAD trial reduced the risk of developing depression, and physical function benefited as well:

Rubin RR, Wadden TA, Bahnson JL, Blackburn GL, et al. Impact of intensive lifestyle intervention on depression and health-related quality of life in type diabetes: the Look AHEAD trial. *Diabetes Care* 2014; 37(6): 1544-1553. DOI: 10.2337/dc13-1928. PubMed reference number: 24855155. Free full text.

Collaborative care between specialists and general practitioners can give good results. For example, one trial focused on intensive medication management of depression, heart disease and poorly controlled Type 2 diabetes. Medical, psychological and quality of life outcomes all improved over a year:

Katon WJ, Lin EH, Von Korff M, Ciechanowski P, Ludman EJ, et al. Collaborative care for patients with depression and chronic illnesses. *New England Journal of Medicine* 2010; 363(27): 2611-2620. DOI: 10.1056/NEJMoa1003955. PubMed reference number: 21190455. Free full text.

Antidepressant treatment

In people with poorly controlled Type 1 or 2 diabetes and depression, a year of antidepressant treatment (using the drug sertraline) was more effective in helping depression than cognitive behavioural therapy (CBT), but blood glucose levels did not improve with either treatment:

Petrak F, Herpertz S, Albus C, Hermanns N, et al. Cognitive behavioural therapy versus sertraline in patients with depression and poorly controlled diabetes: the Diabetes and Depression (DAD) Study: a randomized controlled multicentre trial. *Diabetes Care* 2015; 38(5): 767-775. DOI: 10.2337/dc14-1599. PubMed reference number 25690005. Abstract only.

Website and forums

www.diabetes.co.uk ('The global diabetes community').

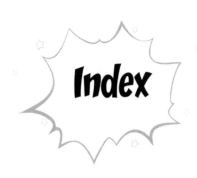

Index

Index

Index